AROMATHERAPY

VIKTOR BLEVI
And
GRETCHEN SWEEN

Illustrated by Sandra Rediger

AVON BOOKS 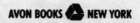 NEW YORK

Note: Natural medicines are generally safe and effective. But, despite every effort to offer expert and well-tested advice, it is not possible for the authors to predict an individual person's reactions to a particular treatment. *Always* refer to the cautions given in Part II under specific plant essences before using any of the treatments recommended. If in doubt, consult a qualified doctor, physician or practitioner of natural medicine. Neither the publisher nor the authors accept responsibility for any effects that may arise from giving or taking any type of natural medicine, or any other related remedy or form of treatment, included in this book.

AVON BOOKS
A division of
The Hearst Corporation
1350 Avenue of the Americas
New York, New York 10019

Copyright © 1993 by KnowIt Publications, Inc.
Cover illustration by Susan Johnston Carlson
Published by arrangement with the author
Library of Congress Catalog Card Number: 92–93929
ISBN: 0–380–76429–6

First Avon Books Trade Printing: April 1993

AVON TRADEMARK REG. U.S. PAT. OFF. AND IN OTHER COUNTRIES, MARCA RE-GISTRADA, HECHO EN U.S.A.

Printed in the U.S.A.

OPM   10   9   8   7   6   5   4   3   2   1

Contents

Part I:
An Aromatic Overview

Part II:
The Essential Guide to Essence

Contents

~~~~~~

Appendixes

Introduction

THIS BOOK IS MEANT TO SERVE AS AN INTRODUC-
tion to the practice and philosophy of aromatherapy. It is
not a medical textbook. However, the research and professional opinion catalogued here should foster a better understanding of a health practice that has recently been
getting a great deal of attention. I hope that it clarifies the
basic parameters of this artistic science/scientific art and
that it might encourage readers to investigate further the
various holistic approaches to health and beauty currently
resurfacing in the Western world.

Generally speaking, aromatherapy is the use of fragrant,
natural substances in health care, beauty aids, and even
food. It is not limited to the use of plant oils, although
these little bottles of aromatic liquid magic were probably
what stimulated the reader to sniff out this book. The role
of essential oils is discussed at length in this volume (in
particular, see Chapter 2); however, the term "aromatherapy" can even describe what happens if you rub a hand
through a rosemary plant and then inhale the fragrance
emanating from your palm: For a moment, your head clears
and your spirits lighten. The aromatherapy discussed in this

book runs the gamut from simple acts whereby natural fragrance can be integrated into everyday life to far more scientific procedures involving commercially prepared essential oils.

Aromatherapy and holistic medicine in general have become exceedingly popular. But aromatherapy, properly understood, is more than a fashionable, fringe phenomenon. I feel the resurgence of interest in holistic, natural health care reflects two significant cultural changes currently taking place. First, we are witnessing the breakdown of the mechanistic view of nature that has dominated our culture since the seventeenth century with the rise of empirical science. Environmental issues and health crises (such as widespread cancer, cardiovascular diseases, and famine) are challenging the centuries-old assumption that man is entitled to enslave Nature, bring her under the yoke of human reason, in order to harness her secrets for man's "superior" ends.

Just as we are starting to recognize the inadequacies and dangers inherent in modern science's imperialistic attitude toward nature, our culture is beginning to question an attendant assumption: that the human body is best understood as a marvelous machine. Growing dissatisfaction with the methodology, expense, and often frightening side effects associated with traditional medicine is causing Westerners to become more receptive to alternative, environmentally and humanistically respectful health-care practices, of which aromatherapy is one.

Instead of viewing the human body as a machine, holistic health-care practitioners see the body as a complex natural system. They treat the body as an interconnected hierarchy of functions, including the central nervous system. It is understood that the human body is highly sensitive to its environment, and this environment is comprised of a vast variety of stimuli—psychological, dietary, sensory, hereditary, and cultural. This view is somewhat foreign to modern science, which functions through classification, objectification, and specialization. Aromatherapy defies the boundaries associated with modern science and mind-body dualism in general.

I believe one reason why aromatherapy and other forms of natural medicine have become appealing is that they suggest a means for human beings to reconnect with the rest of the natural world. Although our own experience may suggest that humankind has always behaved as the enemy or conqueror of nature, not all human cultures have been organized in ways that encourage such an antagonistic, anthropocentric (or human-centered) worldview. Furthermore, our own culture hasn't always emphasized the divisions rather than the connections among experiences and categories of knowledge. Only in recent centuries have human civilizations made distinctions among science, art, and religion. Historically, many of the most famous scientists and philosophers were also poets: Aristotle, Francis Bacon, Goethe. Furthermore, Nostradamus, the great healer of plagues, and Isaac Newton viewed their scientific work as a religious activity. The rigid disciplinary boundaries among these various aspects of human experience were largely products of a mechanical worldview, joint products of empirical science and the industrial revolution. The mechanical worldview enabled human beings to place themselves above the rest of the natural world and see nature as lifeless, readily malleable, and irrational. Once cut off from the rest of nature, the human enterprise of industrial expansion, which seemingly required the exploitation of natural resources through mining, excessive irrigation, and unrestrained deforestation, could and did take place. The mechanical model enabled man to dissect himself in addition to his cosmos, breaking himself and his world down into smaller and smaller parts, increasingly losing sight of the whole.

But the sharp differentiation among disciplines (and human experiences) has informed the way we live for less than two hundred years—about as long as technology has been our reigning sovereign. During this time fields like aromatherapy have been left out in the cold because they fail to fit neatly into any specific category of learning. However, once again the ruler with which truth, knowledge, and value is measured seems to be changing. Many people are attracted to ideas and practices that take into account the whole person as well as his or her environment. In part, this stems from the increasing public awareness of the failure of technology to solve all of our problems. In fact, most people are conscious of the danger into which unrestrained industrialization and the squandering of natural resources has placed our planet. And, as mentioned above, we have seen the breakdown of the technological model, which views the human body as a machine, in modern medicine. Consumer dependence on pharmaceuticals in the United States is exorbitant, but the pitfalls of that dependence are becoming increasingly apparent. The debilitating effects of the overindulgence in synthetic antibiotics is well documented. They can trigger allergies, destroy white blood cells, and create nervous conditions comparable to epileptic fits.

Sometimes progress requires that we take a few steps "backward," that we reexamine the wisdom of the past in a new light. Often we affirm that the truths of other eras were best abandoned; other times we discover that valuable wisdom has been needlessly undermined or discarded. The latter appears to be the case with many of the health and beauty treatments now placed under the rubric of aromatherapy.

Aromatherapy, as it is now called, has a long and venerable history dating back to the most ancient human civilizations. Although its contemporary form is supported by the resources of scientific investigation, modern laboratories, and a more refined knowledge of horticulture and human physiology, there is a strong continuity between the aromatherapy practiced today and its antecedents.

Neither the ancients nor contemporary proponents of aromatherapy perceive a radical distinction between the treatment of mind and body. The aromatherapist emphasizes that treatment should always take into account the whole person: his or her physical and mental health, personality, and his or her perception of life, self, and sickness. The physical, psychological, and spiritual are seen as deeply interconnected. Aromatherapy acknowledges and honors the human feedback loop uniting experience, worldview, and well-being.

Many current medical findings are now substantiating the aromatherapists' claim that we are most often stricken by infections when our resistance is diminished by depression, stress, feelings of low self-worth, and the kinds of physical neglect that tend to accompany these psychic states. Potentially harmful bacteria may exist in the body for long periods of time without engendering disease or infection. Chemical imbalance in their environment (namely, our bodies) can trigger the bacteria to rear their ugly heads. Chronic fatigue, allergies, sexual and reproductive dysfunctioning, asthma, low-level anemia, and

5

other ailments have all been linked to psychologically in-
duced chemical imbalances, imbalances that are exacer-
bated by the poor diet and lack of exercise that often
accompany sustained emotional distress. Thus, it seems that
emotional stability is a strong defense against illness. Furthermore, an optimistic attitude on the part of both healer
and patient can be a weighty factor in prompting speedy
recovery. Optimism is a function of knowledge; we all experience fear and doubt when we are kept in the dark. But
when mutual trust, respect, and information are exchanged
between both parties participating in the healing process,
the patient experiences far more confidence in his or her
ability to get well. The nature of aromatherapy is such that
the patient is able, and even required, to play an active
role in his or her own healing.

Aromatherapy, as this book hopes to explain, involves
using plant essences to heal and beautify. A host of different
plants are utilized by various doctors and therapists, and
this book by no means covers them all. The ones included
here have been selected to offer the reader a sense of the
scope of the field. Furthermore, I have tried to focus on
those essential oils that are most readily available and about
which there has been a considerable amount of research.
It should be noted that, although the evidence about the
healing properties of plants is quite impressive, aromatherapy works best when used in conjunction with other
therapies, a whole foods diet, regular low-stress exercise,
massage, and a strong sense of self-worth.

This book is divided into two major sections. The first
section, "An Aromatic Overview," is broken down into
eight chapters, each focusing on one aspect of aromatherapy. Some of the questions I have tried to address in

the book's first section are: "What is aromatherapy and how does it work?"; "What kinds of substances are involved?"; "What are the roots of aromatherapy?"; "How scientifically valid is this practice?"; "What are some common aromatherapy treatments?"; and "What other practices are associated with aromatherapy?"

The second section of the book, "The Essential Guide to Essence," includes a brief account of thirty-two plant essences commonly used in aromatherapy. Each plant entry contains a general horticultural description of the plant followed by an explanation of its unique aromatic qualities. In most cases I have included a little history about interesting uses to which the plant has been put in earlier times. Next, each entry lists the medicinal properties ascribed to the plant and some of its applications. Finally, each entry concludes with a comprehensive list of each plant's effects.

At this juncture, I would like to confess that I researched and wrote this book as a means for satisfying my own curiosity. While authoring a text on the nature of beauty and cross-cultural beautification practices, aromatherapy was one of the topics I stumbled across. Initially skeptical, I was intrigued by how much casual media attention this seemingly "fringe" practice was receiving. As I pursued my research I gradually discovered that this ancient-contemporary practice is relevant to many areas in which I am more readily conversant: holistic philosophy, the cognitive sciences, and interdisciplinary scholarship. As a teacher and Ph.D. candidate in an interdisciplinary humanities program, I am deeply interested in phenomena where the boundaries among art, science, philosophy, and spirituality intersect and overlap. As I hope this volume demonstrates, aromatherapy constitutes the site of such an intersection. Furthermore, as a fervent amateur organic gardener, the opportunity to study the literature associated with aromatherapy has prompted me to bring aromatic practices into "my own backyard," so to speak. I have felt stimulated and nurtured by the results.

Finally, I must stress that this book is written neither by an expert nor for an expert readership. Keep in mind: All self-treatment has its limitations. Persistent, serious health problems should always mandate consultation with one's health practitioner. Much of the information amassed here is speculative, reflecting opinions—not unqualified truths —articulated by experience aromatherapy practitioners who themselves have encouraged a cautious attitude toward their work. Certainly, pregnant women and children under the age of two should refrain from using herbal medicines and essences without a doctor's careful supervision. If aromatherapy is taken seriously as a cure, it should also elicit caution. Medications of any kind are serious business. And if the very premises of aromatherapy are correct, nature has always exhibited more power than modern man has given her credit for!

Part I

An Aromatic Overview

1
Aromatherapy Defined

"Physicians might (in my opinion) draw more use and good from odors than they do. For myself have often perceived, that according unto their strength and qualitie, they change, and alter, and move my spirit, and worke strange effects in me: Which makes me approve the common saying that invention of incense and perfumes in Churches, so ancient and so far-dispersed throughout all nations and religions, had an especiall regard to rejoyce, to comfort, to quicken and to rowze and to purifie our senses."

MONTAIGNE

Modern research has confirmed Montaigne's earlier suspicions. Aromatherapy, as the word implies, is a contemporary therapeutic process that utilizes fragrant substances. However, the name is somewhat of a misnomer because, although the chemical composition that accounts for the unique aroma of a plant essence is critically linked to its medicinal properties, aromatherapy is not simply a matter of scent. Plant essences, and many other parts of plants, are used by aromatherapists in capsules, bath and massage oils, skin ointments, compresses, infusions, douches, mouthwashes, foods, alcoholic solutions, and, of

11

course, inhalations. In every case, these substances are completely natural and are derived chiefly from plants. This book focuses on the use of essential oils, or essences, derived from a plant's leaves, wood, or flowers; however, there are mentions throughout of ways in which plants—especially herbs—can easily be used aromatherapeutically as they are found in nature, especially in the kitchen or bath.

The plants employed by aromatherapists each exhibit special characteristics and general tendencies and these qualities are described in the "Essential Guide," which constitutes the second section of this book. But because aromatherapy dictates that each individual be seen as an individual, part of the aromatherapist's responsibility (and craft) involves matching unique plant essences with the specific needs and body chemistry of each person. In aromatherapy, there are no sure formulas, only greater probabilities, based on grounded intuitions, empirical perceptions, extensive botanical and physiological knowledge, and a more systemic approach to healing.

Still, the curative success claimed by aromatherapists is nothing at which to turn up one's nose. Remedies have been applied to a variety of ailments—physical, psychological, and cosmetic—ranging in degree from near-fatal to fairly superficial. Dr. Jean Valnet, a French physician, is one of the most eminent experts to integrate aromatherapy and herbology with traditional medicine. He and other European physicians have published case histories that trace the cure of cancer, tuberculosis, diabetes, and other extremely serious and "hopeless" health problems using only aromatic plants and essences, phosphoric acid, magnesium, and liver extracts. On the other end of the spectrum, casual experimenters have found safe, quick, and economical treatments for everything from acne to migraines.

However, the philosophy behind the therapy is what is, perhaps, its most dramatic contribution to contemporary medicine. Aromatherapy is fundamentally holistic. The connection underlying disorders, the whole problem—not just the symptoms—is addressed. The aromatherapist views the body as an integrated system, not as a collection of discrete parts. All illnesses are perceived, to some extent, as manifestations of the mind. In other words, physical disorders are not viewed in a vacuum but are seen as concomitant with mental states.

In many ways, aromatherapy is related to the practices of herbology, homeopathy, and natural medicine, as well as to some environmental movements. All of these practices are concerned with nonviolent intervention upon the human body or upon our larger environment, the earth itself. They all reflect the perception that long-term, global, site-sensitive choices are the best ways to promote health, happiness, beauty, and personal dignity.

Aromatherapy, related to (and frequently overlapping) the other holistically oriented practices named above, has its roots in a time when art and science were not viewed as disparate enterprises but two sides of the same coin. Present-day aromatherapy nurtures a neglected link between "folk medicine" and modern technology. Folk and traditional medicines have claimed to derive many healing properties from plants. However, until relatively recently, we did not have the scientific knowledge to substantiate the earlier wisdom. Aromatherapy resurrects and seeks to legitimize much ancient wisdom, first by taking it seriously and then by fortifying it with methodical testing.

Contemporary technology allows us to account for the successes of numerous ancient home remedies the modern pharmaceutical age had dismissed with condescension. Extensive experimentation has revealed the presence of hormones and antibiotic properties in many plants and essences. Meanwhile, an increase in information concerning the complications that result from the use of aggressively synthesized chemical medications has made some otherwise skeptical researchers more receptive to the natural therapies provided by essences.

The roots of aromatherapy date back to antiquity. Plant essences play a significant role in the medicinal and cosmetic lore of ancient Egypt, China, Greece, Rome, and India—where it is still religiously followed, even in hospitals. Essential oils have been used in the creation of perfumes for centuries. But aromatherapy was transformed into a comprehensive psychological, physical, cosmetic science in the twentieth century through the work of a French chemist, Rene-Maurice Gattefosse, and his followers.

Aromatherapy and its attendant philosophy definitely appear to be gaining both recognition and popularity. *The Natural Food Merchandiser*, a leading trade publication in the natural-food industry, recently reported that sales of herbs in natural-food stores in America rose from $105 million in 1982 to $160 million in 1989; sales of herbal medicinal capsules went from $55 million in 1985 to $87 million in 1989. Some natural aromatic remedies are already available in national convenience stores and drugstore chains! And Americans are actually behind the times. The Chinese have been using herbal remedies continuously for thousands of years, and they are still widely distributed there through pharmacies, hospitals, and clinics. In France alone there are hundreds of practitioners of aromatherapy. Throughout Europe, some medicinal plant essences outsell medical pharmaceuticals. Reputedly, ginseng root is the "drug" of choice in Germany and France.

Aromatherapy involves a collaboration with, not a conquering of, nature. There is no equivalent in conventional medical practice for the preventative therapies attainable with plant essences. They are not invasive, as are Western drugs and injections, such as flu season vaccinations, which prevent future illness by subjecting a healthy person to a host of harmful and unpredictable side effects.

Patients who have suffered from the unexpected side effects that often follow treatment with pharmaceuticals are now taking more initiative with their health, transforming their diets, exercising, and embracing natural remedies, among which plant essences play a significant part. Although the medical community at large has yet to endorse aromatherapy, the benefits proved by practical experience have been sufficient to earn the respect and curiosity of many people. Common sense, at least, reinforces the connection between fragrance in health and beauty. Just as we associate beauty and goodness, we assume that pleasant scents suggest value while we experience unpleasant scents as inauspicious. Although a beautiful face does not always mean that a beautiful human being exists behind it, the intuition that scent reflects the underlying structure of an entity is scientifically sound. The scent of a substance is a function of its molecular structure; unpleasant smells often indicate the impending collapse of the entity, as when organic matter is in the process of decomposing. The pleasant smells produced by nature are frequently signs of health and healing as well as beauty. After using plant essences, one manifestation of the cure is a subtle change in body odor; eliminations from the body begin to emit the aromatic fragrance of the healing plant! Understood thus, natural perfumes are not superficial cosmetics but symbols of the beauty and health that permeate one's being.

2

What Are Essential Oils?

ALTHOUGH AROMATHERAPISTS UTILIZE PLANTS IN a variety of ways, the most common application involves the use of small quantities of plant essences—several drops, depending on the patient, the ailment, and the treatment. The drops of plant essence are placed in capsules, diffused through lamps or humidifiers, mixed in alcoholic elixirs, used in skin ointments, or rubbed directly into the skin.

Plant essences, also called essential oils, are highly concentrated, volatile, vegetal extracts. "Volatile" means that the oil evaporates readily. Therefore, if the oils are not stored properly they quickly lose their active constituents, including the properties that produce their scent.

Virtually all plants used in aromatherapy, especially herbs, flower blossoms, and resinous woods, have a fragrance in their natural state as a complete organism. However, the fragrance of any given essence is both qualitatively and quantitatively different. For example, if you were to rub your hand over a basil plant and then sniff your hand, you would be greeted with a unique smokey, licoricelike scent; however, the essence of basil is much more piercing, resembling peppermint mixed with thyme. In general, the aromatic properties of plants are formed in the leaves' chloroplasts, the sites of photosynthesis. There the essence combines with glucose, a crystalline sugar, to form glucosides. From the leaves, the glucosides are carried throughout the plant, just as nutrients are carried through the human body via the bloodstream. The fragrance of the whole plant is a function of the essence that permeates its leaves, flowers, or bark, but once the essence is removed and concentrated it is greatly intensified.

The term "essence" has another meaning, though, one that will be helpful in understanding the role of essential oils in aromatherapy. In general, "essence" refers to the unique, intrinsic quality that makes something what it is. The "essence" of a human being has been defined by different philosophies as self, soul, mind, or consciousness. In any case, the essence of something is its core—where the truth about that entity is contained. The word "essence" encapsulates what we can mean by words such as "personality" or "life force." In plants, the essence is the site of each plant's uniqueness. No two oils smell alike. And although some oils share affinities with other oils, each has utterly distinctive properties.

Aromatherapy focuses on how plant essences are beneficial to human beings. But essential oils initially play an important role in the biochemistry of plants themselves. A plant's essential oils are like its hormones. In flowers, fragrance assists in the fertilization process by attracting insects. Essential oils catalyze and control biochemical reactions, distribute messages between cells in response to stressful situations, and regulate production and renewal of cells. Furthermore, when the sun's heat causes essences to evaporate from its surface, essential oils protect a plant from parasites and infection by bacteria and fungi.

Depending on the plant, essences may be taken from flower petals, leaves, roots, or the wood. In many plants, the oils are even discernible in tiny droplets: for example, in the leaves of rosemary, the flowers of lavender, the bark of cinnamon, the rind of oranges, and the resin of myrrh.

Essential oils are removed from plants during specific seasons and even at specific times of day. One reason plant medicine may have fallen into disrepute in the past is that people have failed to comply with some basic requirements of procurement and preservation. In each case, the part of the plant in question must be picked before the plant itself is fully developed; leaves are picked just as flower buds appear and flowers are picked before they are fully blooming. Flower buds and the bark from resin-producing trees are procured in spring; fruits and shrub bark are picked in fall; roots can be obtained in the spring and fall; and tree bark should be picked in winter. All plants should be gathered in dry weather early in the morning before the sun has begun to effect the essence's evaporation.

Essences must be extracted from a plant with care and precision. They are removed through a variety of methods, again dependent upon the kind of plant involved. Some are removed through pressing, tapping, separation using heat, by solvents, by enfleurage, and by distillation. Distillation is the most common method of procurement.

The characteristic aromas of herbs, flowers, and spices

are a result of the molecular structure of the plant's essence. Furthermore, essences are analogous to the blood of a person. Like blood in a human body, the essence of a plant is the vital stuff necessary for life, but it is not synonymous with the whole human being. Essences are not the whole plant in miniature, instead they possess a complete, organic structure of their own. Like blood, essences will lose their life force if not properly preserved, and like blood they retain characteristics of the source from which they are derived. The essence is the most fragile and elusive part of the plant but, paradoxically, it is more potent and its impact on the human body is more dramatic than that of the whole plant. This is why essential oils are always used in small doses and are often diluted in other liquids.

Most essences are clear, although some are distinctively colored: cinnamon essence is a beautiful reddish brown, chamomile is blue, and juniper is a yellowish green. Most weigh less than water, although some, such as garlic and cinnamon, are heavier. Essences tend to be soluble in alcohol, ether, and fixed oils, but insoluble in water. But, like water, essential oils are absorbed quickly into the skin. As the vast majority of the human body is made of water, our bodies are quite receptive to essential oils and transport them expediently to internal organs. Inside the organs, the powerful vitamins and enzymes contained in essential oils are processed.

The science of chemistry has enabled us to break organic substances, such as essential oils, down into their component parts for identification and separation. The chemical composition of essences is complex, but they commonly contain alcohols, ketones, terpenes, aldehydes, and esters.

Dr. Taylor of the University of Texas at Austin has demonstrated that essences contain more previously unexamined compounds than all chemists in the world could analyze in a thousand years!

The component parts of essential oils—specifically, the vitamins, hormones, antiseptics, and antibiotics they contain—account, to an extent, for their curative action; but these constituents do not entirely explain their success in beauty and health care. The first modern scientist to practice aromatherapy, Gattefosse, was the first to demonstrate that "the whole is greater than the sum of its parts." Essential oils work holistically; the complex, global structure of an essence working as a whole will always be far more effective than the individual components of an essence applied separately. This is why synthetic oils that have the exact same chemical components fail to provide the same results.

In studying aromatherapy, it is important that one understands two crucial characteristics of essential oils: first, their intense concentration; second, their ephemeral quality. The merit of essences is paid for: It takes a lot of plant to derive a little oil. The percentage of oil present varies widely from plant to plant. Here are some of the average yields from 100 kilograms of a sampling of aromatic plants.

Eucalyptus	3 kilograms
Hyssop	400 grams
Juniper	500 grams to 1.2 kilograms
Lavender	2.9 kilograms

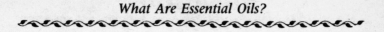

Rose	0.05 kilograms
Sage	1.6 to 2 kilograms
Thyme	200 grams
Ylang-ylang	1.6 to 2 kilograms

In addition to their high concentration, essential oils are very delicate. Without proper preservation they will quickly evaporate. Essences should be preserved in well-sealed colored glass containers away from light. If these precautions are not taken, the following will occur: oxidation, polymerization (when compounds form with different properties from the original), and resinification (when the oil dries out and thickens).

The concentration and location of essences also vary from one specific plant to the next, even among the same type of plant. Differences in soil conditions, climates, and methods of cultivation will affect the quality of a plant's essential oil. This is why oils from certain parts of the world are more valuable than others; certain varieties of essential oils are more potent and more intensely aromatic. (Ceylonese cinnamon and Bulgarian rose oils are two examples of premium essences.) In addition, the chemical composition of the essence within an individual plant is continuously in flux. In a single plant, the essence will change with the seasons and even with the time of day.

The evaporation rates of essences are also variable. Patchouli and sandalwood oils are the most dense and slowest to evaporate, while eucalyptus and orange blossom oils are the least concentrated and most volatile. All other essences exist somewhere in between. There are three general categories. The denser oils, like sandalwood, tend to be resinous oils. These are long-lasting and useful against chronic conditions; they are often used as fixatives when blending several oils or as bases in expensive perfumes. The middle-weight group includes most spice oils and some herbs like lavender; these are particularly good for aiding digestion and stimulating metabolism. The lighter oils, including rosemary, juniper, and sage oils, are the fastest to act; they are excellent for countering lethargy, melancholy, and physical and psychic fatigue. The aromatherapist and perfumer use knowledge of evaporation rates to insure balance and durability in mixtures.

Essences exhibit an impressive range of medicinal properties, some of which can be observed in action at the level of the whole plant. However, one must keep in mind that, although an essence usually has the same properties—be they antiseptic, antispasmodic, astringent, or whatever—as the plant from which it comes, the chemical constituents are typically quite different. Just as the fragrance of an essence is more intense than the fragrance of the whole plant, the action of the essence upon the body, especially the emotions, is more pronounced because the instantaneous effect on the nervous system is greatly magnified.

In addition to their medicinal role, aromatic oils are used in food and toiletries. In foods, they are used as natural flavoring in sodas, jams, and confections; for example, peppermint, cinnamon, and anise essences are quite common in food products. In cosmetics, they are often incorporated into perfumes and used less often as an active ingredient in toothpastes, shampoos, body lotions, and bath products. And it is not only in aromatherapy that the medicinal properties of plant essences are tapped outright; a number of patented products, such as hair tonics, ointments for skin disorders, and antiseptic creams, utilize essences. Actually, anytime you use a health or beauty care product containing plant essences you are practicing a simple form of aromatherapy. As I mentioned in the introduction, aromatherapy is not simply a matter of smell, or at least "smelling" as it is commonly understood. This fact will be elaborated in Chapters Four and Seven.

3

A History of Aromatherapy

I⊤ IS OBVIOUS THAT WE HUMANS HAVE USED OUR SENSE of smell to survive as long as we have had noses. We have used our sense of smell to find food and to avoid eating spoiled or harmful food.

Prehistory

During the Neolithic period, six thousand to nine thousand years ago, humans discovered that fatty oils could be extracted from certain plants, such as the olive tree, through the process of pressing. These oils were used to protect the skin from the sun, to keep the hair manageable, and for cooking. Many researchers speculate that the cuisine of this period entailed cooking with aromatic herbs. It is likely that scented oils were discovered at this time.

The Ancients

Egypt

The Egyptians were the first sophisticated aromatherapists. Fragrant scents pervaded all aspects of Egyptian life, especially among the nobility. Some of the first "aroma-therapists" were priests, who administered scented unguents as part of elaborate religious rituals. In Heliopolis, the city established for the worship of the sun god, Ra, incense was burned three times daily. As the day progressed, the blend of incense became more complex; kyphi, the incense burned at sunset, was a mixture of thirteen essential oils and raisins. Although I know of no accounts that explain the specific rationale behind this practice, the ritual itself reflects the strong association between spirit and fragrance, between religious transcendence/spiritual healing and aromatic experience.

The first aromatic practice that was implemented exclusively for healing was probably fumigation, a process whereby plant oils, later called "incense," were burned until smoke engulfed a room occupied by the patient. We now know that the burning of incense in close quarters was an important practice in ancient Egypt and Babylon. Fumigation was viewed as the best means to combat evil spirits (which were thought to manifest themselves in the form of nervous conditions). And in spite of the smoke, it was believed that the intensely gratifying fragrances purified the air and lungs. In some other cultures too, including many African civilizations, menstruating women were placed in shelters where the air was thick with incense smoke. This practice probably reflects a variety of conflicting attitudes toward the phenomenon of menstruation: It was viewed as magical, frightening, unclean, and meriting protection.

The Egyptians believed that beauty was a spiritual necessity, an essential part of pleasing the gods. They also believed that they would enter the world beyond the grave in their earthly body. As a result, they thought it was important to go to the grave in style, equipped with cosmetics and finery—including their cherished aromatic oils. Alabaster vessels, designed for housing scented oils and dated between 3000 and 2000 B.C., have been unearthed from Egyptian tombs. The twelfth dynasty, which began around 2000 B.C., is famous for its obsession with beauty. Many cosmetics were developed during this time: black kohl used as mascara and eyeliner, vivid blue and green eye shadows, red ocher to tint lips and cheeks, henna to dye the hair and stain the fingernails, and a variety of unguents, ointments, perfumes, and fumigants made of aromatic oils.

Egyptian beauty and health rituals became increasingly complex. Quite unlike Westerners, the ancient Egyptians recognized the therapeutic and preventative value in bathing. The Egyptians knew that baths keep the skin healthy, smooth, and moist while relaxing tired muscles and nerves (a fact Europeans took centuries to embrace). Aristocratic women would regularly bathe three times a day: a cold bath in the morning, a tepid bath in the afternoon, and a hot bath before retiring. The hot bath was always scented and followed by a massage with cedarwood or cypress oil. In addition to softening and preserving the skin, scented oils were used on the hair and the gums. Egyptian men would place a cone of solidified unguent from resinous plants on their heads and let it melt slowly during the course of the day, enveloping the body in rich perfume.

Cedarwood oil was the favorite of the Egyptians. This is why they annexed part of the great Lebanese cedarwood forest into their empire. In addition to using the oil for preserving the complexion during life, they employed it in their mummification process. Apparently, Egyptian doctors were also able to anesthetize patients with a full-body maceration of plants and copious amounts of cedarwood oil.

India

The Egyptians were not the only early culture to appreciate the power of aromatics. In India, where the wisdom of aromatherapy is still practiced religiously, even in hospitals, references to the use of essences have been found in Vedic writing that dates back several thousand years. Numerous references in the Vedic texts and the Kama Sutra, a spiritual book that includes sacred poetry as well as extensive instructions for lovemaking and beauty care, suggest that sandalwood oil was the special favorite of the Indians.

China

The ancient Chinese had a very refined understanding of aromatics, in terms of both medicinal and cosmetic properties. In the oldest known medical document, composed in China in 2000 B.C., the emperor Kiwang-Ti writes about the healing attributes of pomegranate, opium, and rhubarb. The Chinese eventually classified their remedies in terms of yin (the "feminine" principle, associated with wetness, darkness, passivity, and cold) and yang (the "masculine" principle, associated with dryness, light, motion, and heat); a Chinese healer always strove to restore a balance of these two opposite elements in the patient. Some of the most exotic essences, such as jasmine and cinnamon, originated in China, which Europeans only discovered during the Crusades.

Greece

The ancient Greeks also made elaborate use of essential oils on hair, skin, feet, jaw, eyebrows, knees, and so forth. The pantheistic religion of the Greeks ascribed divinity to all plants, so they viewed plant essences as pure spirit. Perfume was also said to be heaven-sent via a nymph attending Aphrodite, the goddess of love. The Greeks developed an elaborate system for anointing different parts of the body with different types of scent.

Rome

The Romans, if anything, were more elaborate than the Greeks in their use of aromatic oils. Several major cities had their own perfume districts. Some of the preparations traded there were very expensive, but the *unguentarii*, the Roman perfumers, never wanted for customers. At the public baths—the centers of Roman cultural life—men would luxuriate in steam baths fumigated with aromatic oil or bathe in a hot tub doused with oil and follow up with a massage with more fragrant oils. The Romans used essential oils and perfumes on virtually everything: their bodies, hair, clothes, furniture, the walls of their homes, and their flags.

Middle Ages

Europe

After the Fall of Rome, Europe began to lose its pleasant smell. The Romans, their knowledge, and their intoxicating fragrances fled to Constantinople. The Byzantine empire became awash with fragrance.

Meanwhile, strides toward the science of chemistry were under way in Arabia. The process of distillation was discovered. It was first implemented on the rose. Rose water became one of the prize commodities of the East. With the Crusades, numerous exotic essences were imported to Europe, including some which had been lost since the fall of the Roman Empire.

Although Medieval Europeans lost touch with the wisdom of personal cleanliness, they continued to be attracted to aromatics. The great plagues of the Middle Ages were largely a result of the horrendous absence of hygiene; interestingly, one of the few effective measures taken to combat the plague was fumigation with pine oil. Aromatics were the most powerful antiseptics available at the time. Those who worked with aromatics, especially the perfumers, were mostly immune to the plague.

Europeans did not set up their own perfume-manufacturing outfits until the twelfth century. Initially, manufacturers relied on imported essential oils and Oriental formulas. It wasn't until the end of the thirteenth century that European perfumers began to create their own scents using indigenous plants such as lavender. By the fourteenth and fifteenth centuries, information about the medicinal use of herbal oils was beginning to be recorded and distributed. There are numerous extant manuscripts from this period containing recipes for health and beauty care treatments involving essential oils along with many unsavory ingredients such as dried flies, urine, and bat dung!

The Sixteenth Century

William Turner, the sixteenth-century herbalist, is often referred to as the father of botany. He classified herbs and illnesses in terms of degrees of hot and cold. In some ways, his thinking was comparable to the medieval system of four humors, wherein the different elements—earth, wind, fire, and water—were associated with different parts of the body. Turner created herbal remedies to correct physical illnesses—for him, manifestations of either too much internal heat or cold. That is, he used essential oils with "cooling" properties, such as peppermint, to treat illnesses of excessive heat, like fever.

The Seventeenth Century

The seventeenth century inaugurated the golden age of herbal medicine. Most of the essential oils considered important today had been isolated by this time. This was the age of the great physician and herbalist Nicholas Culpeper, who used plant essences to heal. He published several significant books on herbs and essences in addition to a beauty manual called *Arts Master-Piece, or the beautifying part of Physick* (1660). The latter is full of recipes, the vast majority of which call for aromatic resins, herbs, oils, or waters, and is still influential among contemporary aromatherapists. The book is dedicated "To All Truly Vertuous Ladies."
And these ladies needed all the help they could get. . . .

The Eighteenth Century

In the eighteenth century, bathing was still frowned upon; it took two more centuries to convince most Europeans—nobility and commoners alike—that bathing was not only worthwhile but a health necessity. Aromatics were seen as a favorable alternative to bathing. Society ladies who viewed bathing as dangerous and immodest would douse themselves in aromatic oils and paint their faces instead of washing them!

The Nineteenth Century

By the nineteenth century, scientific procedures and technology for procuring and testing plant essences had become more refined. In 1882, William Whitla published his *Materia Medica*, wherein he discusses the known constituents and properties of twenty-five different essences. But as the science of chemistry became more sophisticated, herbs were more often abandoned in lieu of synthetic drugs that seemed to act more powerfully. Apothecaries began to exclude essences from their inventory, keeping only those useful as flavorings and carminatives (substances that cause the expulsion of gas from the alimentary canal to relieve colic or intestinal pain). At the same time, the European perfume industry experienced steady growth, using natural oils almost exclusively. In southern France, around the area of Grasse, the cultivation and extraction of essences became (and remains) a big business.

The Twentieth Century

In the earlier twentieth century, a chemist named Rene-Mauricé Gattefosse began working with essences in relation to the cosmetic industry. During an explosion that resulted from an experiment gone awry, one of his hands was badly burned. Almost without thinking, he soaked it in neat lavender oil. However, he claims not to have been surprised when the burn healed with exceptional speed, leaving no scar or indication of infection. After this episode, he proceeded to focus his research on the healing properties of plant essences. Gattefosse was the first to use the term "aromatherapy." He published his first book on the subject in 1928, followed by numerous papers and other books, mainly relating to therapy using essential oils.

Since Gattefosse, there have been many others who have made significant contributions to the field of aromatherapy. Dr. Jean Valnet, a French physician who began his career as an army medic, remains the leading contributor. His work has brought the most legitimacy to the practice. He has published numerous books and articles specifically addressed to the French medical community wherein he documents his extensive success in treating a dramatic range of illnesses with natural medicines and, specifically, essential oils. In print, he has always referred to his medical methodology as aromatherapy and phytotherapy (treatments using plant substances). He has written, lectured, and broadcast widely on his findings. In spite of the obvious innovation of his contributions to the field, he has modestly pointed out that during World War I aromatherapy—that is, the use of essential oils for healing—was fairly common in some military and civilian hospitals. Lacking supplies, the hospital staffs turned back to some of the other remedies that had been abandoned in favor of "modern" cures. Working in hospitals during the war, no doubt inspired by Gattefosse, Valnet was given the impetus to pursue this field that had intrigued him since his childhood.

Another important figure in aromatherapy research is Marguerite Maury, the Austrian biochemist and two-time winner of the Prix Internationale d'Esthetique et Cosmetologie (an international prize awarded for exceptional scientific contributions to cosmetics research). She developed the foundation of a medicinal/cosmetic therapy based on massage.

Essential oils and plants were universally the dominant health and beauty aids from their first discovery until the late eighteenth century. Aromatherapy was then gradually superseded by chemically manufactured drugs. Aromatic essences were belittled, underrepresented, and demystified in order to elevate the synthetic chemical industry, which was seen as more rigorous and quantifiable and, therefore, a better complement to modern science. However, the tradition of aromatics never entirely faded. Like the mummies in the Louvre—the corpses the Egyptians preserved with injections of cedarwood oil—latent knowledge of aromatics has survived for thousands of years. And now, we are seeing a resurgence of interest in this artful science of scent with its whole-body approach to healing.

4

How Aromatherapy Works

THE SENSE OF SMELL IS THE MOST SENSITIVE, DYNAMIC, and efficient system in the human body. Impulses are carried directly from receptor cells housed in the nose up to the brain. But in order to really understand how scents can enable healing, it is important to grasp some theoretical principles.

A Swiss physician and alchemist, Paracelsus, wrote in the sixteenth century: "All is poison, nothing is poison." With this statement he was referring to the paradoxical aspects of many things. Aside from medieval alchemists, the ancient Greeks as a whole were far more aware of this phenomenon than we are now. Their very language reflects an understanding of how substances can cause opposite and complementary effects. For example, in classical Greek there is a single word that means both "medicine" and "poison." Understanding aromatherapy is contingent upon understanding this principle: There are no monolithic treatments, just as there are no absolute, singular definitions that can be ascribed to entities in our perspectival cosmos. To put this observation colloquially: One person's garbage is another person's treasure.

Aromatherapy works by correcting imbalances, yet the application of one particular kind of essence does not produce one kind of result. All essences have a range of therapeutic actions. Likewise, all ailments addressed by aromatherapy can be treated by several oils. Furthermore, the quantity of a dose will have everything to do with the reaction it induces; with some essences a small dose may stimulate the nervous system while a large dose will have a sedative effect. In either case, an essence (or blend of essences) with the appropriate intensity will promote the reestablishment of equilibrium within the body, a truce between opposite forces.

It is imperative that certain conditions be met in order for essences to have more than a superficial effect. The plants from which they will be derived must be grown in an appropriate location and picked at just the right time. When plants are used in their natural form they must be dried and stored carefully in order to preserve their power. And they must always be used with discrimination and knowledge. Commercially produced essential oils deserve the respect proffered any drug, which entails reverence for their power as well as their benevolent curative properties; they should be stored safely, protected from extreme temperatures, and used only in recommended dosages.

There are many methods for administering essential oils. They can be ingested in the form of capsules (which contain straight oil) or drops of the oil alone. Drops are often mixed with honey water or alcohol—the latter because essential oils are readily soluble in alcohol. Anywhere from five to thirty drops may be in order depending on the essence, the illness, and the general constitution of the patient. Externally, essences may be used in their pure form, diluted for general or localized bathing, added to a humidifier, combined with other essential oils to treat the skin directly, combined to form soapy emulsions, inhaled from a bottle, mixed with water or white vinegar to create liniments, douches, and enemas. Furthermore, aromatherapists administer creams, sprays, lotions, and massage oils that contain essential oils as the active ingredient. Because these oils in their natural form are so highly concentrated, they are always used in tiny doses.

A vast number of odoriferous substances can be used medicinally. If one is interested in exploring aromatherapy, the best place to start is in the kitchen. The use of freshly cultivated aromatic plants and seasonings in cooking—garlic, onions, rosemary, thyme, savory, cloves, and so forth—will produce noticeable benefits: clearing the head, lightening the spirit, and promoting healthy digestion. Dried herbs and flowers kept in the house and stored in closets, and aromatic herbs growing on a windowsill will variously purify the air, repel insects, and create an environment more conducive to work and play.

Because of their purity, essences are rapidly diffused. Whether introduced through the nose, mouth, skin, rectum, or vagina, or intravenously or intramuscularly, essences quickly permeate the body. As a result, essences applied locally can have large-scale, general effects. Not only do essences possess curative properties in their own right, all essences increase the efficiency of other treatments through the speedy elimination of waste and toxins from the tissues.

Another reason essences are capable of discouraging the spread of infections and toxins has to do with their acidic pH value and their constituent antiseptic agents. Acidity combats the rapid proliferation of microbes inside the body. The primary constituent of clove essence, for instance, is eugenol, which has not only antiseptic but also fungicidal and local anesthetic properties. Dr. Valnet reports that medical researchers in West Germany have even developed a clove-based general anesthetic.

Aromatherapists often prescribe the administration of essential oils to the skin through massage or baths. These oils quickly pass through the layers of skin, circulate in the blood, and are then eliminated through the lungs and kidneys. In the process, organs benefit from the essences' disinfectant, stimulant, or antispasmodic properties.

In human embryos, the nervous system (including the brain) and the sense organs are formed from the ectoderm at the same time as the skin. After birth, these remain closely linked—that is, substances, or "data," introduced through receptors in the skin will be processed quickly via the central nervous system, relying on important feedback from all the sensory systems. It is as if our nose, eyes, and ears are located all over our bodies.

The justification for external applications of essential oils is interesting. Doctors have become increasingly aware of how porous the skin is. Many substances, after being applied to the skin, will quickly be absorbed and transported all over the body. As a result of this knowledge, many doctors are now administering drugs through skin patches in lieu of hypodermic needles. However, the message underlying this revelation is that we should be cautious about the quality and quantity of substances we rub into our skin. In terms of personal-care products such as deodorants, bath scents, and skin lotions, one should seek out the purest, most natural products available, or even investigate making one's own from herbs and essences. Be wary about the use of the words "pure" and "natural" on product labels, however. There are no federal regulations controlling the use of these terms and they often appear on products that are actually loaded with synthetic materials.

The real secret to the success of aromatic essences is their organic nature. Unlike many synthetics, they are more than an "on-off switch," simply stimulating or sedating. They normalize and reestablish balance. They are sensitive to the specific body chemistry of individuals while promoting adaptability in the body at large. At the same time, each essence has an affinity with certain emotions, certain parts of the body and mind, and individual taste. Oftentimes the scent a person finds most pleasing will prove to be especially beneficial for that particular individual. However, I do not mean to imply that going around sniffing bottles of pleasant-smelling oils can cure serious ailments. As a matter of fact, too much random olfactory stimulation can, quite simply, produce a headache or even nausea. But it is worthwhile to keep in mind that the nose, as the external end of the olfactory system, connects directly to the brain. Therefore, on a certain level, the nose has an intuitive sense of what the body needs!

I will clarify the relationship between the chemical constituents of natural medicines (specifically, essential oils) and human body chemistry in the following chapters.

5

Aromatherapy As Science

"Many things will be reborn which have long been forgotten."

HORACE

WITH THE INITIAL RISE OF MODERN SCIENCE AND THE pharmaceutical industry, the use of aromatic essences fell from grace. In part, this was because objective scientific analyses failed to yield explanations to account for the healing power of plants. Our infatuation with quantifiable, statistically based knowledge caused us to turn away from centuries of traditional, empirical evidence that demonstrated that plants can perform a wide variety of medicinal operations.

The magic contained in essences eluded modern scientific investigation until recently because the structure of essential oils is extremely complex. Even now that much scholarship has embraced the subject, we are still unable to reproduce the exact structure of a single essence. Artificially reconstituted oils have revealed the chemical constituents of the oils, but their odor and therapeutic action are always somewhat inferior to their natural counterparts.

The recent realization among scientists that human beings cannot quite compete with nature in this area has enabled them to appreciate the inherent sophistication of essential oils. Science and folk traditions are finally beginning to reintegrate, and energy and funding are being channeled into discovering just how and why essential oils affect the mind and body.

Many individuals and cultures have noticed that body odors and perfumes trigger emotional responses. We now know that body odors are produced by the apocrine glands, which develop fully only in puberty. These glands release through sweat all kinds of information about a person: his or her diet, hygiene and personal habits, health, emotional state, and sexual receptivity. Every person has an odor as unique as a fingerprint. This smell is further influenced by our heredity, occupation, and even our mood.

Contemporary research has confirmed that unpleasant odors can actually cause a person to feel physically ill or produce sexual dysfunctions such as temporary impotence; pleasant odors can instantly counter general debility and raise a person's spirits. Smells can elicit memory recall. As a matter of fact, the sense of smell and memory are so closely linked that sufferers from Alzheimer's disease lose their ability to smell in tandem with their loss of memory.

The nature of smell remains a compelling subject for contemporary scientific research. At Yale University's Psychophysiology Center, researchers are investigating how certain smells can stimulate alertness and others reduce stress. Tests conducted by the University of Cincinnati have demonstrated that the introduction of fragrances into the atmosphere of a room increases work efficiency.

At the Monell Chemical Senses Center in Philadelphia, a large research complex, vast numbers of scientists are employed in studying the chemistry, psychology, and the curative role of smell. In addition, Monell is interested in examining some of the more unusual features of our most elusive sense. Their concerns are similar to those associated with aromatherapy: how body scents can be used to diagnose disease, how they influence social behavior—subliminally and consciously—and how we are able to identify different smells. Furthermore, they are concerned with how a person loses his or her sense of smell, a problem that afflicts only one out of every two million people but that can prove both life-threatening and life-deadening. Without the ability to smell, one cannot detect gas leaks, unseen fires, or putrefied food; in addition, many of the pleasures associated with being human disappear—the "taste" of good food and wine, the fragrance of flowers, the scent of the people one loves.

Researchers at Monell and elsewhere have determined that we are not entirely different from other biological creatures in the ways that we are influenced by scent. But although science is demonstrating that this tendency is shared across all levels of the biological world, even within our own species some responses to scent vary a great deal from one individual to another. Different scents combine to produce different, and sometimes conflicting, sensations, and these vary from person to person. Practitioners of aromatherapy are especially concerned with the relationships among scents and the effects of different scents on different body chemistries, instead of analyzing them in a vacuum, as was the practice formerly when performing conventional research.

Although aromatherapy remains outside the mainstream of medicine in the United States, numerous eminent researchers, biologists, pharmacists, and doctors have authored articles and books on the healing properties of plants and essences. In France especially, aromatherapy is quite well respected within the medical community at large. And because the world has always turned to the French for innovations in the art of beautification, aromatherapy has been embraced by many cosmeticians and therapists in spas throughout Europe.

In general, scientific analysis of essences and the nature of scent is confirming that aromatherapy is nothing to sniff at! Many pure oils contain natural preservative properties that retard the development of fungus, yeast, and bacteria. Some oils activate the drainage of certain wastes or draw them directly out of the skin. There is significant evidence that aromatherapy has been used successfully to retard aging, treat migraines and arthritis, heal acne, stimulate drainage of lymph glands (which leads to the disintegration of cellulose and lowers blood pressure), and deal with a multitude of other ailments.

Every essence has unique properties, but all essences tend to stimulate the production of leukocytes. Leukocytes are small, colorless cells in the blood that aid in the body's defense against infection by destroying alien microorganisms. This is why even the most casual use of essential oils constitutes sound preventative medicine; they are natural, risk-free antibiotics.

Investigation by the scientific community of the claims of aromatherapy and other natural medicines has even raised questions about the curriculum in conventional medical schools. Medical students spend shockingly few hours studying diet and nutrition. Furthermore, holistic medicinal practices like aromatherapy are teaching that healing doesn't just happen at the microscopic scale—the medic must begin to consider the whole person in prescribing treatment. The tendency within the medical community to break the human body down into smaller and smaller systems is proving to have serious limitations. Proponents of aromatherapy, homeopathy, and natural medicines urge us to look at the human body "systemically," that is, as a complex, integrated unit where everything we put in—air, food, cosmetics, drugs, ideas, and so forth—influences the body's performance. Thus, not only is science enhancing the long folk tradition of aromatics, aromatherapy is altering the way we view contemporary science.

6

Natural Versus Synthetic Substances

BEFORE DELVING INTO THE CENTRAL THESIS OF THIS chapter, I would like to take a moment to clarify the term "natural." At the very least, "natural" means "found in nature." By this definition it is safe to say that plants are natural. The essence derived from a plant is also natural, although the process by which it is removed from the plant is basically a human invention. To be precise, the separation of essential oil from plants is in a sense a "naturally" occurring phenomenon, as when the sun causes the essential oil on the petals of a rose to evaporate. But in terms of the essential oils used in aromatherapy, human technology has refined the process significantly so that a part of nature is isolated and then translated into another, more readily usable form—namely, a concentrated liquid. In general, we call the latter practice "science."

During the past few centuries, science, or rather, scientists, have gotten better and better at separation and translation. Essential oils themselves have been broken down into their constituent parts. The capacity to dissect has then enabled scientists to "copy" some of nature's original handiwork. These "copies" are known as synthetic chemicals.

Although they sometimes bear structural similarities, natural and synthetic substances are perceived as occupying opposite poles. Synthetic substances—in cosmetics or medicine—are of human invention; they are derived by combining two or more chemicals into a single compound. Natural substances, as the term implies, are used as they are found in nature. Of course, all biological entities are comprised of chemicals. All fruits and vegetables, for example, are broken down into chemicals within the digestive system. All chemical substances are simpler or more primitive in structure than biological entities. However, organic substances, such as the essential oil from the leaves of a eucalyptus plant, have far more complex structures than chemical compounds, such as eucalyptol, the chief constituent of eucalyptus essence, which can be reproduced synthetically. Both eucalyptus essence and its constituent, eucalyptol, are found in nature. But eucalyptol working within the structure of the essence is more effective as an antiseptic than it is when isolated and combined synthetically with other chemicals. The bottom line is that, on this front, nature is the better designer: Her work is too difficult to duplicate—synthetic simulations lack the dynamism of their natural antecedents.

Some real confusion occurs when manufacturers use the word "natural" to suggest botanicals when they aren't really in the product. The term "natural" is rendered still more confusing because it is often used interchangeably with "organic." But "organic" specifically refers to a substance derived from something once living. There are beneficial natural ingredients derived from inorganic substances, such as clay.

Furthermore, some terms we now hear frequently are "organic gardening," "organically grown," and "organic fruits and vegetables." For the uninitiated, this term seems like just a fancy redundancy designed to enable merchants to charge more for their tomatoes. In fact, organic gardening is a specific process whereby produce and grains are grown without the use of pesticides, herbicides, or any synthetic chemical substances. Instead, plants are grown using exclusively natural substances like microbial-rich soil and compost; fertilizers like bat guano, seaweed kelp, fish emulsion, and earthworm castings; and pesticides are replaced by beneficial insects such as green lacewings, trichogramma wasps, and ladybugs. Foods that are organically grown are certainly more "natural" in that they were produced with the unadulterated resources of biological (as opposed to inorganic) nature. Most plants from which essential oils for aromatherapy are derived are organically grown.

Unfortunately, it is still somewhat difficult to find products designed for wide-scale distribution that are entirely natural. Synthetic substances are less expensive and require less time to process. About 60 to 70 percent of the composition of most expensive perfumes is synthetic. Inexpensive perfumes are entirely synthetic.

Although synthetic fragrances are more cost-effective to produce, they lack the complexity of natural essences. But after years of domination by the chemical industry, the production of cosmetic products is going back to basics: natural botanical essences, oils procured from fruits, flowers, herbs, and vegetables. Many lines of hair-care and skin products (like Bio-Logics, initiated by Richard Stein of New York City) are now learning from history and are reintroducing natural ingredients like nettles, chamomile, and rosemary into their products. These products are generally not the ones advertised as "natural" in regular supermarkets; many of those mass-produced commodities still have the same chemical components with 5 percent natural extracts added, largely for fragrance. The genuinely wholesome and environmentally sound products are available in specialty and health food stores and many salons.

Most shampoos advertised on television and sold in supermarkets contain lathering agents like sodium lauryl and ammonium lauryl sulfates. These synthetic substances were first introduced into shampoos because people were convinced that without lather, hair wasn't really getting clean. In fact, these chemicals dry out the scalp and strip hair of its natural protein coating. As a result, people turn to conditioners.

Most conditioners coat hair with an oily residue that gives the impression of body but actually has no real effect on the hair itself. Moreover, the filmy layer attracts dirt. Thus, a day later, one needs to wash the hair again; the cycle begins again, significantly weakening the hair and drying the scalp over time. If one uses all-natural hair rinses, it is only necessary to wash one's hair twice a week. Furthermore, one's natural hair protein is fortified and the scalp is lubricated and nourished.

Another difficulty arises from the fact that, although many cosmetics must include a list of ingredients on their packaging, some items most of us would classify as cosmetics are actually considered over-the-counter drugs by the FDA. These items include: fluoride toothpastes, antiperspirants, deodorants, deodorant soaps, and dandruff shampoos. Manufacturers of these goods are not required to list ingredients, nor are any cosmetic manufacturers required to test their products for safety. Usually this kind of testing is done only after harmful effects have been reported.

Side effects from synthetic cosmetics, as with all chemical drugs, are cumulative. Synthetic chemicals are not as easily processed by the body as natural substances are. They gradually amass within one's system, meanwhile creating a feedback relationship within the body that distorts and intensifies a person's reaction to the chemicals in the initial product. After using a product for an extended period of time, seemingly without any problem, one can "suddenly" perceive a serious reaction. But the reaction is not really sudden. The cycle of short-term fix followed by slight degeneration just finally breaks down altogether. The body announces "Enough is enough," and produces a symptom. This can happen with everything from mouthwash to deodorant.

To take one specific example, some of the ingredients recognized as harmful found in antiperspirants and deodorants include: aerosol propellants, dyes, ammonia, formaldehyde, ethanol, glycerin, and the generic "fragrance." During the past decade, more than eight ingredients commonly found in these products have been banned by the FDA or voluntarily removed because they had proved injurious to consumers. The most common complaints are skin irritations, frequently quite serious. As consumer awareness rises and demands for safety increase, it makes better economic sense for the manufacturers of cosmetics to become more conscientious about their consumers and the world in which these consumers live.

The trend toward health consciousness in the beauty business is beginning to filter down to the medical world as well. As far back as 1973, during a "Hospital Week," a group of international doctors discussed the harmful effects of aspirin on the stomach. In a major study, 51 percent of digestive hemorrhages were traced to aspirin consumption. In *Cold Cures*, Michael Castleman lists a multitude of side effects that commonly result from America's "drug of choice": aspirin.

Americans consume more than twenty billion doses of aspirin a year, adults averaging one hundred tablets per year. However, this seemingly benign household staple is known to upset the stomach and cause ringing in the ears, and in large doses can impede our blood-clotting mechanism, obstruct liver function, contribute to anemia, and increase the risk of birth defects; and when taken by children who are already mildly ill can sometimes lead to the fatal Reye's syndrome, which debilitates the liver and brain. Other common antiinflammatory pharmaceuticals that have posed health problems include phenylbutazone and the derivatives of cortisone.

Unlike synthetic drugs, which have a violent, generic action on human beings, regardless of the individual's unique constitution, essences work within the system to restore its natural balance. Essences work with the natural healing process of the body, whereas chemical drugs, like antibiotics, kill bacteria indiscriminately—the innocuous and valuable bacteria as well as the detrimental. Furthermore, the body becomes easily habituated to synthetic drugs, gradually requiring an ever-increasing dosage to achieve the same results. However, one never really builds up a tolerance to natural essences. Synthetic chemicals create artificial swings in the body—a "high," or respite from pain, fatigue, infection, odor, or other symptom, followed by a rebound effect. Gradually the body generates an immunity to protect itself from these unnatural swings, necessitating ever larger dosages or applications of the synthetic substance in order to produce the original "up" phase of the swing. Natural substances do not induce dramatic swings nor are they difficult for the body to assimilate and process; therefore, there is no reason for the body to generate an immunity to them. Thus, to suggest that one can become inured to the tools of aromatherapy would be like proposing that one becomes habituated to organically grown vegetables, clean air, or personal hygiene.

Although a body can become inured to the toxins in synthetic drugs, this protection is short-lived. Eventually, the body's defense mechanisms become exhausted and the system malfunctions. The once "miraculous" success in treating a range of conditions attributed to many antibiotics and synthetics has not held up in the long run.

Antibiotic mania is being challenged right and left recently. Antibiotics are now recognized as catalysts for allergies. In fact, allergies are most common in countries wherein there is widespread use of antibiotics in the general population. Because it has been so overly and indiscriminately used, many people in the United States have grown sensitized to penicillin. Reportedly, antibiotics have renal toxicity and cause nervous disturbances, sometimes comparable to epileptic fits. In addition, the use of antibiotics sets up a vicious cycle in our immune system: The drug kills bacteria, immunity develops, new kinds of bacteria emerge, one turns to another kind of antibiotic, and so forth.

After expending a considerable amount of energy processing isolated chemicals, the body can develop numerous serious health problems. The strain can cause liver damage, faulty metabolism, anemia, cirrhosis, gall bladder problems, and a fall in white blood cell count. If taken by pregnant women, many synthetic drugs, will damage the fetus and create birth defects.

Psycho-drugs represent another dangerous area of synthetic consumption. The vaguely termed "tranquilizers" and "nerve stimulants"—or more basically, "uppers" and "downers"—are severely overprescribed and overused in the United States. Paolo Rovesti, an Italian professor who worked with Gattefosse, aromatherapy's "founding father," has studied the effect of essences on the psyche. He writes: "According to sociologists and neurologists the salient characteristics of our age are those of anxiety and depression, and material proof of this is available in the even higher figures shown for the consumption of tranquilizers and stimulants. It is well known that disturbance and toxicosis can be caused by these products if taken regularly." Rovesti goes on to explain that, used in the proper dosages, aromatic essences are completely harmless because they do not produce any of the side effects such as trembling, memory loss, stupor, hyperactivity, chronic nausea, and appetite loss associated with psychotropic drugs.

Many of today's medical practitioners focus on suppressing symptoms rather than seeking the cause of the complaint. But the body creates its symptoms with great wisdom. A symptom usually points to exactly what the body needs in order to heal: vomiting because the digestive system has been polluted and requires purging; or headaches because of straining one's physical or mental capacities, suggesting that some relaxation and release of tension is in order. Millions of research dollars have been applied to the task of finding a cure for the common cold. A single drug has yet to be found because researchers have isolated over a hundred different strains of the illness! But the answer is really quite simple when put in general terms: A cold needs heat. This heat can be procured in the form of an essential oil whose action is warming, such as black pepper or clove essences. Likewise, a fever requires something like eucalyptus oil, which is cooling.

As early as 1960, Brun, Kalb, and Possetto wrote in *Presse Medicale*: "[T]he abundance and repetition of administered drugs, particularly antibiotics, together with the abuse of stimulants means that more and more often patients are in a highly complex state of sensitivity which peculiarly modifies their individual reactions to therapies which might otherwise be considered innocuous." Because natural medicines do not pose these long-term problems and can even heal the consequences of destructive cycles of habitual synthetic drug use, they merit serious consideration as an alternative, if not complete substitute, for synthetics.

7

The Sense of Smell

"Smell is a potent wizard that transports us across thousands of miles and all the years we have lived. The odors of fruits waft me to my southern home, to my childhood frolics in the peach orchard. Other odors, instantaneous and fleeting, cause my heart to dilate joyously or contract with remembered grief. Even as I think of smells, my nose is full of scents that start awake sweet memories of summers gone and ripening fields far away."

HELEN KELLER

THE SENSE OF SMELL IS THE MOST SENSITIVE AND among the most efficient systems in the human body. It is remarkably precise, even though it may not be as precise as a dog's, which is over a million times more sensitive! Still, the average person is capable of identifying thousands of different scents.

Our distant ancestors relied upon their noses a great deal. Their sense of smell was far more refined and sensitive than ours. Today, the combination of underuse, a polluted atmosphere, a heavily mucus-producing diet, and cigarette smoking have sorely degenerated our sense of smell.

But even considering the shameful way in which we have abused and neglected our olfactory sense, machines have been unable to replace us in sniffing capacity. In all cosmetic control laboratories, biochemical research centers, and some lucky police departments, there is a machine running continuously; this delicate, expensive piece of machinery implements a process known as chromatography, a method whereby the different constituents of a liquid are distinguished in order to discover its composition and detect any inconsistencies. In cosmetic and drug laboratories, the machine is used for quality control. However, in every laboratory, working alongside the supposedly "infallible" machine, is a person known as a "nose." This man or woman will sniff the vapor given off by the liquid and check it against the machine's graph. In all circumstances, the "nose" knows best. It is an individual in a very human body who is equipped to determine whether or not the machine-generated data are correct. As was mentioned earlier, our noses do become sensitized to smells, but this is only after continuous exposure to a single scent. Thus, a person working as a professional "nose" couldn't sit around smelling the same fragrance over and over; she or he needs intervals between each testing. But as a rule, the olfactory mechanism of a "nose" is so sensitive, and his or her olfactory memory so refined, that he or she is able to detect subtle variations without too much effort.

Despite the keen sensitivity of our nostrils, we often find it difficult to describe specific scents in words. Likewise, scientists' attempts to explain and categorize the mechanisms of the olfactory system are somewhat feeble. We do know a few things; for example, the ability to smell is carried out by microscopically small organs, receptor cells with long hairlike structures called cilia embedded inside a mucus

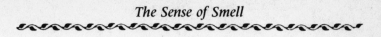

layer of the cells. There are between six and twelve hairs per cell. Odors enter the nose as minuscule droplets that must be soluble in the mucus in order to be detected. Once the droplets are diffused they trigger impulses that are then chemically transmitted to the brain. The hairs are direct projections from the nerve cells that transmit to the brain. The other end of the cell leads directly to the olfactory bulb in the brain. As a result, olfaction involves far more immediate interaction between neuron and stimuli than any of the other senses. The olfactory nerve is connected directly to the brain via the nose; this is the only direct gateway to the brain. This is why olfactory stimulation can have an immediate effect on the nervous system—a fact that the research of aromatherapists has sought to reinforce.

Our olfactory nerves connect directly with the limbic system, the older, reptilian part of the brain. The limbic system is not under our conscious control. It regulates behavior associated with our primal drives such as hunger, thirst, and sex. The limbic system directly influences the digestive and reproductive systems and our emotional responses to sensory experience. Thus, the process of olfaction is not an intellectual experience nor is it easily subjected to analysis. Our "understanding" of smell is the product of images and associations.

Daniel McKenzie, author of *Aromatics and the Soul* (1923), argued that what we think of as the sense of smell is actually a division of labor between two mechanisms; because they work simultaneously we experience them as a single phenomenon. He claimed that one type is chemical and operates in the manner described above; in other words, molecules must in fact be inhaled. The second type is vibration and does not depend upon the physical presence of molecules. The latter is the best explanation science has generated to date to explain how some creatures manage to pick up scents at great distances.

In 1967, J. E. Amoore published an article in *Nature* magazine presenting his findings on the relationship between certain shapes and odors: Round molecules smell of camphor, disc-shaped ones of flowers, and wedged-shaped molecules smell like peppermint. Some researchers have proposed a connection among odor, color, and sound perceptions—all of which have healing potential. As E. Douek, author of *Perfumery: The Psychology and Biology of Fragrance*, points out, "anosmia" (the inability to smell) is usually accompanied by depression, which is often severe. This is because when one loses the sense of smell what we commonly think of as "taste" is lost as well, making a serious dent in our knowable world.

Blindfolded and with a stopped nose, one would be unable to tell the difference between milk, lukewarm black coffee, and red wine. The pleasure we experience from eating is largely thanks to the olfactory system. As a matter of fact, digestion begins with the nose. The pleasing aroma of food causes the secretion of digestive juices in the mouth. The better our food smells the more readily digestible it is.

Numerous ancient civilizations, such as those of Egypt and Greece, were acutely aware of the fact that body odors and perfumes activate emotional responses. The aromatic lore of these cultures tells us that inhalations of jasmine, basil, or citrus oils relieve depression; a whiff of peppermint oil energizes and sharpens mental acuity; rosemary oil refines the memory.

Different smells combine to produce different, and sometimes even conflicting, sensations. The scent of most perfumes, for example, is quite complicated. While a perfume may smell wonderful in a bottle, it can smell radically different when applied to the skin of different people. It alters as it combines with each person's unique scent. The science of aromatherapy, which attempts to understand scents not only as distinct essences but also in relation to one another, is making important contributions to this field. Aside from its contribution to and rehabilitation of contemporary medicine, aromatherapy has played a part in developing new cosmetic products with organic ingredients.

The human nose is fairly universal in some aspects. We all find some odors distasteful. For example, consider the passage from the first page of Patrick Suskind's 1986 historical novel, *Perfume*, cited below. Suskind describes eighteenth-century Paris where, in terms of stench, the Dark Ages continued to linger in the air. This historically accurate description of Paris is especially amusing in light of the fact that Paris is the city we now associate most strongly with exquisite perfumes:

In the period of which we speak, there reigned in the cities a stench bearly conceivable to us modern men and women. The streets stank of manure, the courtyards of urine, the stairwells stank of moldering wood and rat droppings, the kitchens of spoiled cabbage and mutton fat; the unaired parlours stank of stale dust, the bedrooms of greasy sheets, damp featherbeds, and the pungently sweet aroma of chamber pots. The stench of sulfur rose from the chimneys, the stench of caustic lyes from the tanneries, and from the slaughterhouses came the stench of congealed blood. People stank of sweat and unwashed clothes; from their mouths came the stench of rooting teeth, from their bellies that of onions, and from their bodies, if they were no longer very young, came the stench of rancid cheese and sour milk and tumorous disease. The rivers stank, the marketplaces stank, the churches stank, it stank beneath the bridges and in the palaces. The peasants stank as did the priest, the apprentice as did his master's wife, the whole of the aristocracy stank, even the king himself stank, stank like a rank lion and the queen like an old goat, summer and winter.

By all accounts, Suskind's description is no exaggeration. Western civilization, considered advanced in so many ways, looked on bathing, and hygiene in general, as a suspect practice until well into the nineteenth century. No wonder the big cities like Paris were notorious for their stench!

Aromatherapy is the therapeutic use of pleasant natural substances; however, unpleasant odors also play a role in healing and health, as does our natural response to unpleasant smells in general. The gut-level repugnance we feel in response to certain ugly smells—sometimes emitting from ourselves!—can be a warning signal. Human beings tend to find unsavory those odors that suggest a lack of hygiene, decay, disease, industrial and human waste, and gaseous fumes—all of which are in some way antithetical to our survival. Doctors claim that each specific disease has a characteristic smell; this smell can be understood as part of the warning signal created by the body as a means for seeking help. Doctors of earlier eras had to rely extensively on the smell of perspiration, urine, breath, and feces in making their diagnoses.

As with many things, such as beauty, human beings find it easier to agree about the negative end of the scale rather than the positive. That is, we may be consistent about what constitutes a bad smell, but our feelings about what smells good are more variant. Although there is much discrepancy among people about what kind of food smells good, all humans find the smell of some kind of food pleasant and comforting. As a rule, most people are attracted to sweet, floral fragrances—especially when they are natural.

Ironically, the nose has a more difficult time holding on to pleasant smells. Olfaction is the most dynamic scent; it works quickly and its impact fades after repeated stimulation. If, for instance, one is smelling a rose, the first whiff may strike one as intensely rich and complex, but after sniffing several times in rapid succession, it will seem as if the scent has vanished. This is not because the rose has changed but because our nose quickly becomes acclimated to the scent. Our olfactory perception fades, as if our bodies were telling us, "You've had your share, now don't be greedy!" Unfortunately, this does not happen as quickly with unpleasant odors. This inconsistency suggests that we need more encouragement when it comes to seeking remedies and less encouragement to indulge in sensual pleasures.

To some extent, the degree to which a person finds another attractive is determined by how one responds to that person's natural odor. This unique odor can never be fully masked. Therefore, the best perfumes or colognes are those meant to blend with and complement an individual's personal scent, not one designed to overpower it. While human beings become easily sensitized to their own smell and even that of their fellow humans, we remain subconsciously influenced by the odors of other people. The "chemistry" between people definitely has something to do with a harmonious blend of scents. A study of olfactory characteristics along gender lines demonstrates that by smelling a tube of exhaled breath, 95 percent of both the men and women tested accurately ascertained the sex of the donor. Also, each sex found it consistently easier to identify the breath-scent of the opposite sex.

All of nature seems to be driven by scent. Animals are attracted and sexually aroused by pheromones, aromatic substances secreted by other animals. Mosquitoes are drawn to floral perfumes on human skin. In *The Secret Life of Plants*, Peter Tompkins and Christopher Bird argue that unfertilized flowers exude an especially strong fragrance for up to eight days; if it fails to attract the necessary insects, the flower will wither and die. However, if the flower is fertilized it will cease to emit any fragrance at all within thirty minutes. This evidence suggests that scent plays a sexual/erotic role for plants and insects, as it does for animals and human beings. In a very real sense, nature's nose is what makes the world go 'round.

8

General Methods for Applying Essences

> *"A good name is like a precious ointment; it filleth all around about, and will not easily away; for the odors of the ointments are more durable than those of flowers."*
>
> FRANCIS BACON, *Novum Organum* [1620]

ALTHOUGH THE SPECIFIC APPLICATIONS FOR DIFFERENT essences are elaborated in the next section of this book, this chapter will discuss three general methods for using essential oils. In addition to internal application, essences or blends of several oils are used as health and beauty aids through inhalation, bathing, and massage.

Inhalation

The inhalation of aromatic essences is, as I have discussed, an ancient practice. The Greek physician Marestheus made a career of sniffing different flowers, determining that they had either stimulating or sedative effects. Flowers with a fruity or spicy aroma, such as rose or hyacinth, he found stimulating; he found the fragrance of flowers in the lily family to be calming. Many cultures have used incense in their religious rituals because breathing the perfumed air proved to be both calming and uplifting.

The Latin word *spiritus* means "breath," as well as "inspiration from the gods." The English word "respiration" is derived from the Latin and suggests the deep connection between the sustenance of body and soul. All living cells need oxygen to function; therefore, breathing is indeed the spirit of life. While normal breathing accomplishes the elimination of one third of the toxins produced in the body, inhaling the fragrance of aromatic plants and essences is an expedient way to promote internal health and healing because the chemistry of the fragrance stimulates the digestive system as well.

As a matter of fact, the inhalation of essences can be so powerful that excessive continuous use can cause headaches or nausea; furthermore, the rapid intake of several different essences confuses the nervous system. This does not, however, apply to blended essences wherein a balance has been sought and achieved.

For the refined Victorian lady, smelling salts, or "vapors," were an aromatic necessity. This bottle of essential oils diluted in alcohol was kept around the house and even carried around in a purse; it was used to revive women suffering from fainting spells. Strict Victorian notions of feminine behavior and stifling fashions, such as the mandatory whalebone corset, made fainting a common occurrence among nineteenth-century upper-class women. Although the social circumstances that initially motivated the creation of smelling salts no longer exist, blends of essential oils specifically designated for inhalation are now commercially available to meet different twentieth-century needs. For example, the aromatherapist Daniele Ryman has developed two potions to beat jet lag, one to be inhaled in the morning to keep alert and the other at night to help induce sleep. These particular products, each a blend of twelve different essences, are even being sold in the international terminal at London's Heathrow Airport.

Commercially available diffusers project essences in a thin mist, propelled by air. The following essential oils are useful in diffusers to treat these general disabilities while revitalizing and deodorizing the air and acting as an antiseptic.

- Calming: chamomile, lavender, marjoram
- Stimulating: pine, rosemary, sage
- Purifying: geranium, lemon, oregano
- Clear lungs: eucalyptus, hyssop, lavender
- Antidepressant: cedarwood, frankincense, myrrh

Bathing

Bathing was a central part of social, cultural, and even religious life in numerous older civilizations. The Egyptians, Chinese, Arabs, Greeks, and Romans all developed elaborate bathing rituals. This is because each of these civilizations was aware of the sensual pleasure to be derived from baths as well as their medicinal benefits (such as calming, invigorating, alleviating muscular and rheumatic pains, and revitalizing the skin).

The parallel between the bath and the mythical fountain of youth is not purely metaphoric. Regular and conscientious bathing is both physically and emotionally therapeutic. Benjamin Franklin, who was in many things ahead of his time, recognized this fact. He brought the first bathtub to the United States in the late 1700s largely because he believed he could think more clearly submerged in a tub. In water, much of one's weight is displaced and the blood pressure drops. It has been noted that when water temperature and body temperature converge, the mind experiences a sense of euphoria.

From the moment bathing was brought indoors, people began to amend the water with fragrances. Aromatherapists frequently recommended bathing treatments. The procedure is simple. One usually adds five to fifteen drops of essential oil to a tub and then mixes it so that a light film floats across the entire surface of the water. In general, tepid baths relax and sedate while short, hot baths have a tonic action. Aromatherapists recommend bathing in cool water with eucalyptus or peppermint oil to bring down a fever. Local bathing with scented oils is recommended for healing wounds. Footbaths are especially effective against headaches, colds, neuralgia, constipation, varicose veins, and leg, abdominal, and menstrual cramps.

In baths, a smaller amount of oil is absorbed than with other methods of application. But the oils still have an impact on the nervous system, it is just more subtle. After bathing, use a tiny amount of scented oil to keep the skin supple and to counter the drying effects of soap. Aloe vera gel with a few (literally, three) drops of essential oil is a wonderful moisturizer.

The following oils are recommended for each of the general actions listed. Experiment with blends, but do not exceed a total of fifteen drops per bath. To prevent the possibility of skin irritation use a dispersant such as vegetable oil or a foaming bath gel; mix your essential oils in one of these bases, which are available through most distributors of essential oils.

- Relaxing (evening bath): chamomile, cypress, lavender, marjoram, orange blossom, rose
- Stimulating (morning bath): hyssop, juniper, peppermint, pine, rosemary, sage
- Refreshing: basil, bergamot, cypress, geranium, lavender, lemon
- Aphrodisiac: cinnamon, jasmine, rose, sandalwood, ylang-ylang
- Muscular and rheumatic pains: juniper, rosemary, thyme

Massage

Massage too is an ancient art. It was relished in Egypt and throughout the Orient long before the West had the good sense to hop on the bandwagon. References to anointing are scattered throughout the Bible; the expression "to anoint with oil" actually refers to the practice of massage with scented oils. This passage from John 12:3 is one example: "Then took Mary a pound of ointment of spikenard, very costly, and anointed the feet of Jesus, and wiped his feet with her hair: and the house was filled with the odor of the ointment."

Massage therapy is a central practice in aromatherapy. Massage is still the most efficient and expedient means available for alleviating stress and tension, and, of course, it is far healthier than the tranquilizers some doctors prescribe as if they were vitamins. On the most obvious level, aside from the benefits of deep massage itself, the use of essential oils in massage enhances the experience with the aura of pleasant aromas. But massage is also a productive way to promote absorption of medicinal oils.

The type of massage employed by aromatherapists is a combination of Swedish massage, shiatsu or acupuncture massage, and neuromuscular massage. There are also three forms of aromatherapy massage: back, facial, and whole-body. Whole-body massages usually begin with the back so that the rest of the body is already fairly relaxed before more sensitive areas are addressed.

The masseuse aims to work deeply but without jarring the patient in any way. Deep muscle work is done gently and slowly, causing a minimum of discomfort. The massage process aids in the penetration of the healing oils, stimulates and relaxes the body, and acts on nerves, reflexes, and meridians. Many ailments can be addressed locally by guiding essences to the areas of the body where they are especially needed.

In order for massage to be truly effective, the patient must be relaxed. Likewise, the masseuse needs to feel confident and relaxed. The communication by way of touch is especially important to the healing process; it has both psychic and physical ramifications. But it cannot work without a degree of mutual trust.

Furthermore, massage is not effective unless the skin itself is receptive. The skin needs to provide a clean carrier for the oils traveling through the body. It should not be blocked either from the inside with toxins or from the outside with dirt. The lymph, a body fluid found in vessels between the vertebrae, will not transport oil if it is congested. Unlike blood, lymph does not have a heart to pump it. When it meets with resistance, it stagnates. Lymph stagnation can lead to aching muscles, obesity, cellulite, swollen glands, and other ailments. The most common causes of lymph stagnation—as well as blood toxicity, constipation, and the skin congestion that goes with them—are overeating, poor diet, and lack of exercise. If congestion is a problem, sometimes a short fruit juice fast followed by a change in diet and regular exercise will swiftly clear up the problem. Aromatherapy will work to eradicate the deeper manifestations of these problems.

The protocol for aromatherapy massage is fairly standard. The massage should take place in a warm, comfortable, sparsely furnished space, well lit but without any glaring lights. The patient should lie on a firm massage table or couch so that the therapist can move easily around. The therapist should wash his or her hands both before and after the massage. Once contact begins, the hands should be removed as rarely as possible to insure a steady flow. The masseuse works slowly, searching for pockets of tension. The massage is especially effective when it naturally falls into sync with the patient's breathing. Both participants should avoid conversation, concentrating instead on the healing process.

The basic recipe for creating a massage oil is:

¼ oz. essential oil (total)

12–14 oz. vegetable oil

For dry skin, almond, castor, cocoa butter, olive, and peanut oils are best; for normal skin use corn, cottonseed, sesame, or canola oil; and for oily skin use linseed, soybean, or any nut oil. The following list suggests some essential oils that can be used singly or in blends to promote the actions named.

- Calming: chamomile, lavender, marjoram
- Stimulating: lemon, oregano, peppermint
- Aphrodisiac: cedarwood, sandalwood, ylang-ylang
- Improved circulation: cypress, geranium, thyme

Part II

The Essential Guide to Essence

THE PLANT ESSENCES DISCUSSED HERE ARE REP-resentative, not comprehensive. I have not included every essence used in aromatherapy, nor have I discussed any single essence exhaustively. However, the information should provide a worthy introduction to the art of aromatherapy. All medicinal claims stated here were found in a variety of sources written by practicing aromatherapists.

When taking any essences internally they should be diluted in honey water and imbibed after eating. Recommended therapeutic dosages are as follows:

age	number of drops one oil	number of drops combined oils	number of doses per day	maximum treatment
5–14 years	2	1 each	3	2 weeks
15 and over	4	2 each	3	3 weeks

Usually one week is sufficient to treat most ailments. Chronic cases deserve a doctor's prompt attention. Extremely high doses (ten to twenty milliliters) of some oils can poison the system. However, none of the oils included in this book is toxic.

Because the skin is most often the medium through which essential oils are introduced into the body, before undertaking aromatherapy the skin needs to be relatively healthy to begin with. If your skin is in bad shape, aromatherapy should be preceded by a change in diet, exercise, and a decrease in use of synthetic cosmetics and pharmaceuticals.

Basil

Ocymum Basilicum (Labiatae)

Basil, also known as sweet basil, is an ancient plant from the Pacific Islands. In the sixteenth century, it entered Europe by way of Asia. Early English settlers took the plant with them to the New World. Its name comes from the Greek *basilicon*, meaning "royal ointment."

Basil is a short, hearty bush (although it is grown as an annual in most climates) whose leaves are used in a variety of cuisines. Due to its popularity, it has been much hybridized. Some aromatically significant varieties include African basil (which has a camphorlike scent), cinnamon basil, dark opal basil (which has a heavy perfume appropriate for potpourri), lemon basil, licorice basil, and holy basil (which is sacred in India). The basil most commonly used for medicinal (and culinary) purposes is the variety known as sweet or common basil.

On many levels, this plant activates the senses. Basil shrubs tend to be very exuberant, producing exponential growth in a single season. The most common variety produces little white flowers. The essence is a light greenish yellow. It has a strong, pungent, clovelike aroma that conjures up a lush Mediterranean landscape. The taste of both the leaves and the essence is both bitter and sweet. It has

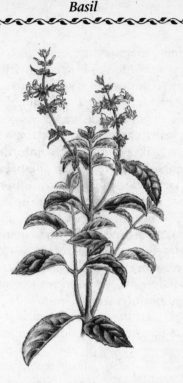

Basil (*Ocymum basilicum*)

the peculiar characteristic of being hot and cold at the same time. Basil essence in a bath will prove both stimulating and relaxing.

The Greeks believed that a basil plant was capable of warding off evil; today in Greece it is still a common custom to keep a pot of basil growing on the front stoop.

The primary properties of basil essence are as a tonic (particularly of the nerves) and as an antispasmodic (first stimulating then calming the activity of the central nervous

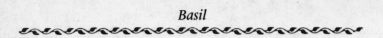

system). Aromatherapists have ascertained that basil is among the best nerve tonics because, when used in appropriate doses, it settles nerves without sedating the patient. It counters mental fatigue, anxiety, painful digestion, spasmodic coughs, migraines, dizziness, insomnia, and sparse and irregular menstruation. Like peppermint, it has a piercing quality that makes it useful for combating sinus congestion. The human digestive system is especially responsive to basil; this fact and its antiseptic qualities make it useful in treating intestinal disorders. Its antispasmodic qualities make it effective against gastric spasms and indigestion.

As for the skin, it invigorates the complexion and can be used moderately as a general toner (five drops diluted in a bowl of warm water). It also works to repel insects, particularly mosquitoes, and has been used in the treatment of insect, scorpion, and snake bites.

- Activates the senses.
- Tonic and antispasmodic.
- Counters mental fatigue and related symptoms.
- Remedy for gastric spasms and other intestinal problems.
- Repels mosquitoes and other insects.

Benzoin

Styrax Benzoin (Styraceae)

Benzoin is a balsamic resin obtained from tropical trees—
also called benzoin—cultivated in Asia. The grayish gum,
streaked with red, oozes out after a deep incision is made
in the trunk of the tree. The red streaks contain the most
aromatic material. The resin is harvested after it has
hardened.

Benzoin is one of the time-honored components in incense and was traditionally burned in sacred ceremonies to
drive away harmful spirits. Its principal component is benzoic acid: a white, crystalline, organic acid obtained by
breaking the essence itself down into its constituent elements. This acid is produced synthetically for commercial
purposes; benzoic acid is a common antiseptic and preservative. The essence of benzoin, which is called a resinoid
(because it comes from tree resin), has a deep auburn color
with the consistency of fatty oils. The fragrance of benzoin
resembles vanilla.

Benzoin is recognized for its capacity to break through
blockages; it eliminates excess mucus, activates circulation,
stimulates urine flow, and unclogs the pores of the skin. It
is especially effective against cold symptoms. It has sedative
as well as antiseptic qualities.

- Antiseptic.
- Purifies and heals skin.
- Eliminates clogging.
- Activates flow of body fluids.
- Remedy against cold symptoms.

Bergamot

Citrus Bergamia (Rutaceae)

Bergamot is a pear-shaped citrus fruit grown largely in Italy specifically for its oil. The tree was named after the city of Bergamo in Lombardy, where the oil was initially brought to market.

The greenish yellow oil comes from the rind of the fruit. It is one of the most commonly used essence oils in the perfume industry, partially because it blends well with almost any other oils. The scent is sweet and tangy, like other citrus fragrances, but it also has an additional floral quality similar to lavender.

Bergamot oil has been used in Italian folk medicine for centuries, especially as a cure for fevers and worms. More recently, medical doctors and aromatherapists have discovered that the antiseptic, antidepressant, and antispasmodic properties of this oil make it useful in a wide range of treatments. Dr. Jean Valnet's case studies demonstrate that it can be used to combat intestinal parasites, colic, and loss of appetite. Others claim that it is useful in douches for combating vaginal infections (leukorrhea and vaginal pruritus). Its disinfectant qualities make it a worthy antidote to bad breath. Furthermore, it activates digestion and disperses flatulence. In moderation, it is a good healing tool against skin disorders such as acne, eczema, and psoriasis— excessive dosages will have the reverse effect. Because bergamot increases the photosensitivity of the skin, it allows one to tan more easily when it is applied in a highly diluted form. However, one should be cautious because it does not protect the skin from the sun's damaging ultraviolet rays.

- Antiseptic.
- Antidepressant, antispasmodic.
- Remedy for intestinal problems.
- Heals skin disorders in low dosages.
- Increases photosensitivity of the skin: Do not use immediately before tanning.

Camphor

Cinnamomum Camphora (Lauraceae)

The camphor tree, native to Japan and China, is a hardy
evergreen in the laurel family. It produces small white flowers in clusters, as well as blood-red berries. However, the
fruit is difficult to harvest because the tree generally grows
twenty to thirty feet before branching. While camphor, the
essence, is found throughout the tree, it takes many years
to develop. Once the tree is at least fifty years old, branches
can be cut. Pieces of wood and the bark are then boiled in
water to extract the essence. The essence, distilled from
steam, becomes solid as the water temperature cools. The
oil is clear and smells similar to eucalyptus.

Camphor has a balancing nature and can counter extreme
conditions in any direction. Therefore, it is particularly
useful in response to extreme and sudden upsets such as
shock, heart failure, and ailments precipitating a rapid
change in body temperature. For example, in treating a
hysterical attack, camphor produces a calming effect;
against a depressive lethargy, it acts as a stimulant. Its most
common function is as a stimulant. In general, camphor
energizes circulation, the heart, respiration, and digestion.
Thus, in addition to the applications already mentioned,

camphor provides a powerful counter to asthmatic attacks, bronchitis, colds, fevers, constipation, extreme diarrhea, pneumonia, tuberculosis, and food poisoning. Because of its antiseptic and antiphlogistic (inflammation-reducing) properties, camphor is good for acne-ridden or otherwise hypersensitive skin.

In a completely different context, camphor is used to protect fabric from moths, because the fragrance repels them.

- Antiseptic.
- Counters and reverses acute and extreme conditions.
- Stimulant.
- Balances hypersensitive skin.

Cedarwood

Juniperus Virginiana (Coniferae)

The cedars are wide-spreading, coniferous trees of the pine family, and have clusters of needlelike leaves, cones, and durable wood. The fragrance from the foliage is so strong that, when one walks near a cedar tree with a breeze blowing, one can smell the tree before seeing it.

Cedarwood oil may have been the first essential oil ever extracted. The Egyptians used it abundantly, particularly in their mummification practices but also as a cosmetic and an insect repellant. King Solomon's great temple was built out of the famous cedars of Lebanon, which are now, unfortunately, very rare. The Lebanese cedar was extremely popular throughout the early civilizations of the Middle East. Because the Egyptians found Lebanese cedars so desirable, they went so far as to annex the great forest into their empire to insure for themselves a plentiful supply of the sacred wood.

Likewise, the American Indians considered cedar trees to be sacred. In Native American lore, it is believed that the Great Spirit who created the universe left a certain mark on all plants capable of providing healing: a pointed top. The cedar tree is one such example. Legend has it that when the Creator made the cedar tree, Grandmother Earth so loved it that she filled its center with her blood, turning the interior red. The Indians were the first to discover that if one burns a cedar smudge as if it were incense and inhales the fumes, it will clear the sinuses, relax the larynx, and calm the soul. Cedarwood essence, used in a diffuser, works as a tonic for the respiratory, glandular, and nervous systems, meanwhile alleviating stress and anxiety.

Contemporary investigation of cedarwood oil indicates that it has an especially powerful effect on skin eruptions of any kind. It combats acne, oily skin, and an excessively oily or dry scalp. Cedarwood oil, in addition to being a insect repellant, relieves itching from insect bites. In some instances, it has been used to treat more serious skin ailments such as psoriasis, dermatitis, and eczema. Too much of this oil, however, will irritate the skin.

~~~~~~

Cedarwood essence, as the name suggests, is extracted from the wood; it is distilled from the sawdust. Cedarwood essence has sedative, antiseptic, and astringent properties.

- Clears respiratory system.
- Combats skin eruptions.
- Relieves itching.
- Alleviates stress and anxiety.

Chamomile

Anthemis Nobilis, Matricaria Chamomilla (Compositae)

The delicate fernlike foliage is strong-smelling, but the dried daisylike flowers are the part of the plant that has been used for centuries to create medicinal teas.

There are several varieties of chamomile, and several "false" ones as well. The apple-scented chamomile known as *Anthemis nobilis* is the variety most commonly cultivated for tea. Several cultures have claimed this variety as their own; thus, common names for the herb are tossed about: Roman chamomile, German chamomile, Hungarian cha-

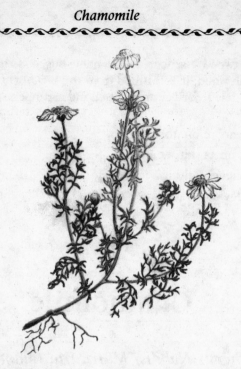

Chamomile (*Anthemis nobilis*)

momile, English chamomile—all essentially the same plant.

Chamomile grows to be about a foot high and abounds in tiny white flowers with yellow centers even in winter. The oil from its flowers is a pale blue. *Matricaria chamomilla* is very similar, although the flowers are smaller and its essence oil is a deep blue.

Chamomile contains the interesting substance known as azulene. It is an intense antiinflammatory agent, named for the blue crystals that form when it is isolated. Azulene is used in a number of pharmaceutical products—such as ointments, soaps, lotions, and creams.

Chamomile

Chamomile was used by the ancient Egyptians to fight fever. Contemporary doctors have recommended internal use of chamomile as a remedy for jaundice, colic, peptic ulcers, urinary stones, and indigestion; external use is suggested to treat burns and skin inflammations of all kinds. Many have noted its pointedly sedative effect; it calms the nerves and eases tension without proving a depressant. Taken internally (even in tea) it is efficacious in treating all kinds of female dysfunctions, especially those that accompany conditions such as PMS; irregular, scanty, or excess menstruation; cramps; vaginitis; and menopausal difficulties. Used in massage oil, chamomile essence will relax strained muscles.

Chamomile is also used in herbal skin-care and hair-care products. Because of its low toxicity, chamomile is good for overly sensitive dry skin as well as for treating acne, commonly associated with oily adolescent skin. It is often used in shampoos and conditioners to lighten or brighten blond hair because of its mild, nonabrasive bleaching properties.

Because chamomile is both gentle and wide-ranging in its therapeutic properties, this herb has been especially helpful in treating children. It can be used to combat all childhood diseases; settle the nerves; counter sleeplessness engendered by nightmares, fevers, or persistent coughs; and ease painful teething.

- Anti-inflammatory agent.
- Calms and sedates.
- Remedies various female dysfunctions.
- Soothes skin.
- Nonabrasive bleach.

Cinnamon

Cinnamomum Zeylanicum (Lauraceae)

The most common cinnamon is from Ceylon, where it is found in the inner bark of an evergreen tree (*Cinnamomum*) of the laurel family. The bark is gathered from new shoots every two years. The bark fragments are rolled into sticks that are sold commercially. In the West, cinnamon plants are grown as ornamentals in greenhouse settings because of the visual and aromatic appeal of their foliage. The essence of cinnamon is distilled from steam when the bark is boiled in water.

Every culture that has encountered cinnamon has found it very alluring. Cinnamon used to be considered a rare and precious commodity, reserved as a special ingredient in feast day preparations. For centuries, cinnamon has been used in pharmaceutical products, as an incense, and as a perfume. Chamberland, writing in 1887, claimed that Chinese and Ceylonese cinnamons were among the most powerful antiseptics known to man. Young children everywhere have discovered how tasty cinnamon is sprinkled with sugar on buttered bread.

Scientists studying the constituents of essential oils now understand why cinnamon has always been so popular: It is a significant circulatory, cardiac, respiratory, and digestive stimulant. Diluted in draughts or syrups, it can be used to counter colds, general disability, difficult breathing, sluggish digestion, diarrhea, impotence, and scanty menstruation.

- Powerful antiseptic.
- Stimulates the general functioning of the body.
- Fights infections.
- May cause irritation and convulsions when used in high doses.

Cypress

Cupressus Sempervirens (Coniferae)

The cypress is a tall, evergreen, cone-bearing tree native to North America, Europe, and Asia. Cypress trees have dark green or gray foliage and a distinctive symmetrical shape. These trees were a favorite planting in cemeteries of the Mediterranean (probably because they were considered sacred on the island of Cypress). Now they are a popular landscape plant, especially in formal gardens. Most often, the cones and branches are used to derive the essential oil through steam distillation.

Cypress oil, with its scent of nuts and dense woods, is similar to pine and juniper oils. The oil from this tree has been used medicinally for centuries; it was popular among the Assyrians as well as Hippocrates, the Greek "father of medicine."

Cypress produces a restraining effect unique among plant essences. Its intense astringent properties enable it to halt bleeding through the contraction of the blood vessels or tissues; thus, it is beneficial against excessive discharges of all sorts, including hemorrhages. It is also an effective regulator of menstruation and female menopause. Some phy-

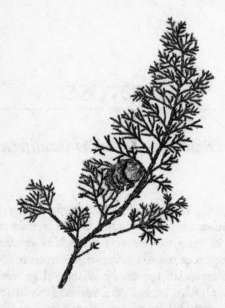

Cypress (*Cupressus sempervirens*)

sicians claim that infusions of the cypress cone—a solution obtained by boiling the cone in water for five to ten minutes—promote scar development and are useful for treating wounds. It has been used externally to treat hemorrhoids, oily skin, and varicose veins. Furthermore, as a powerful antispasmodic, cypress oil is useful against persistent coughs and asthma.

- Astringent, tonic.
- Antispasmodic.
- Stops discharges of all sorts, including hemorrhages.

Eucalyptus

Eucalyptus Globulus (Myrtaceae)

Eucalyptus trees are all intensely fragrant evergreens of the myrtle family and are mostly native to Australia, although now they have been cultivated in many subtropical regions. The eucalyptus, commonly called the gum tree, is probably the tallest tree in the world, reaching up to 480 feet. It bears pendent gray-blue leaves, shaped like little shields, and clusters of pink or white flowers that, as buds, are covered by a cuplike membrane. (This is the source of the tree's name, since *eucalyptos* means "well covered.") The shape of the leaves is especially conducive to retaining moisture (and the essential oil) in the hot Australian climate.

The eucalyptus tree and its oil were first introduced to Europeans in the late nineteenth century by the botanist Baron Ferdinand von Muller. Australian settlers had long used eucalyptus as a folk remedy for colds, fevers, hay fever, snakebites, dysentery, and general aches and pains—among many other ailments; however, they first learned this wisdom from the Aborigines. The Aborigines recognized its pronounced cooling effect on the body, thus its potency for counteracting all kinds of fevers.

There are over three hundred species of eucalyptus. Some varieties are used in medicine, while others with a radically different chemical composition are used in perfumes. The oil is obtained through distillation of the leaves.

Most people are aware of the fact that eucalyptus oil makes an effective mouthwash, inhalant, and chest rub. This is because it is a stimulant, expectorant, and antiseptic substance. A eucalyptus spray can kill off airborne staphylococci. It works to alleviate respiratory and genitourinary tract infections and skin disorders, such as mild burns, herpes, and other eruptions. It is good for throat infections, especially those accompanied by heavy discharges. As an inhalant, eucalyptus can allay exhaustion, lack of concentration, and sinus headaches.

- Relieves aches and pains.
- Cools and soothes.
- Expectorant, relieves respiratory problems.
- Clears sinuses.
- Antiseptic.

Fennel

Foeniculum Vulgare (Umbelliferae)

Hardy fennel is related to dill, anise, cumin, and several other esteemed herbs. Fennel grows wild in much of Europe and on the West Coast of the United States. All varieties of fennel have the characteristic warm, sweet, anise flavor. Anethol is the element of the oil that produces this aroma. Fennel grows four to five feet high and produces clusters of tiny yellow flowers.

Several ancient civilizations valued fennel for its medicinal properties. The ancient Chinese used fennel to heal snake and scorpion bites. They, as well as the Romans, regarded it as a weight-reduction agent. And because of fennel's diuretic property, we can now say that this belief was more than whimsical folklore. However, the Romans also believed that fennel bestowed power and insured good luck on a journey, beliefs that are harder to substantiate with contemporary scientific experimentation! Likewise, during the Middle Ages, fennel was stuffed into keyholes to prevent the entrance of evil spirits.

For centuries, European and American herbalists believed that fennel strengthened sight. On the surface this is deceptive; however, it is true that a very effective wash for tired, red, or strained eyes can be made by boiling fennel seeds in water. The filtered liquid, cooled and transferred to an eyecup, works wonders in a matter of minutes.

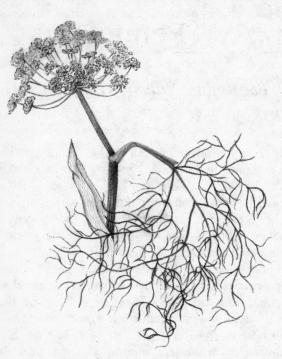

Fennel (*Foeniculum vulgare*)

Fennel seeds are often used to flavor teas, fatty meats, and preserves. However, the leaves are also excellent in salads and sauces. The bulbs of the plant and its stalks (in the manner of celery) are also consumed. Fish grilled with fennel (and lots of butter) is an epicurean delicacy in French cuisine. In addition, fennel is used as a flavoring in many liqueurs, such as Sambucca. The pulverized seeds are said to strengthen the gums while the whole seeds are said to aid digestion. The latter fact is why fennel was brought to the New World by settlers. The essence of fennel is generally obtained through distillation of the seeds.

In 1772, the physician Joseph Miller established that sweet fennel oil is one of the best carminatives, that is, something that helps expel gas from the body. This is because fennel works primarily on the digestive system. It has actually been found useful in treating all digestive and stomach disorders, including colic, flatulence, nausea, vomiting, indigestion, intestinal parasites, constipation, and loss of appetite. Recently, it has been demonstrated that anethol (the chief constituent of fennel essence) greatly reduces the toxic effect of alcohol.

- Treats digestive and stomach disorders.
- Reduces the effects of alcohol intoxication.
- Cleanser.

Frankincense

Boswellia Thurifera (Burseraceae)

Frankincense is actually a gum resin obtained from a variety of small African and Arabian trees. The trees generally produce abundant foliage and white or pale pink flowers. The gum is procured by making a deep cut in the tree, peeling away the bark, and allowing the milky resin to harden for several weeks.

The gum frankincense, also known as olibanum, and myrrh were used by the Egyptians to make the first incense. As an incense, it had several functions. It was used as a sedative, an aphrodisiac, and as a means to drive out evil spirits from the sick. As a matter of fact, the name "frankincense" is derived from the word "incense." The French simply called the substance *encens*, meaning, of course, incense. The English, who acquired it from the French, called it *franc encens*, thus, its modern name.

Ovid, in his *Medicamina Faciei*, a book on cosmetic practices, says that if frankincense is good enough for the gods, mortals ought to find it useful as well. Indeed, frankincense was prized in civilizations throughout the ancient world, so much so that it was perceived as an equivalent to precious gems and gold in bartering. Five thousand years ago, the Egyptians went to great lengths to import frankincense from other parts of Africa. In ancient Egypt it was used not only as incense but as a cosmetic. Supposedly, frankincense was used to create a special facial mask designed to counter the consequences of aging. Its astringent properties have been confirmed and it does seem to have preserving and antiinflammatory potential. In 1922, a pot made of calcite containing remnants of frankincense was found in the tomb of Tutankhamen, who died around 1350 B.C. As a result, we can conclude that this particular substance must have incredible staying power!

Unfortunately, frankincense eventually became one of the most neglected essences, even though it had universal appeal in the ancient world. One explanation for this turn of events is that it has often been compared to myrrh. And although frankincense has a much more pleasing aroma, myrrh is superior in combating mouth ulcers and other inflammations. However, in terms of the psyche, frankincense far outperforms myrrh. It has been demonstrated that the especially pleasing scent of frankincense is excellent for clearing the head, calming the emotions, and alleviating anxiety. Moreover, like other resin essences, frankincense works as an expectorant and has a noticeable effect on mucous membranes.

The essence of frankincense is clear and blends well with a number of other oils including basil, camphor, pepper, and sandalwood.

- Expectorant.
- Relieves stress and anxiety.
- Revitalizes the skin.
- Heals skin and mucous membranes.

Garlic

Allium Sativum (Liliaceae)

Garlic is a bulbous plant in the lily family. The bulb of this
plant, which has a powerful smell, is made up of sections,
called cloves, that are the part of the plant used in aromatherapy. Without doubt, garlic is the most beloved culinary
herb. But while its place in the kitchen is common knowledge, many people are not aware of the fact that it is also
highly medicinal.

   Although the recent move among contemporary American chefs toward native cuisines and indigenous ingredients
has bolstered the position of garlic in this country, older
cultures have had a more heightened appreciation for garlic
than our own. In Egypt, garlic was deified. The builders of
the Pyramids were allocated a clove of garlic each day to
insure fitness and enthusiasm as they toiled at their mon-
umental task. Pliny, the Roman naturalist and writer,
claimed that garlic could cure sixty-one different ailments.
Medieval and Renaissance folklore is filled with homemade
remedies involving garlic. A sachet of garlic worn about
the neck was said to ward off witches and the infectious
diseases they brought with them.

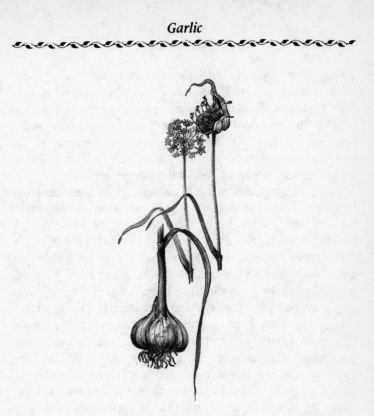

Garlic (*Allium sativum*)

Garlic is indeed a wonder herb. It enhances the immune system and is loaded with nutritional as well as medicinal benefits. Garlic is full of fluorine, phosphorus, potassium, sulfur, and vitamins A and C. The French physician and aromatherapy expert Dr. Jean Valnet recommends the following for breakfast as a general preventative: two raw chopped cloves of garlic mixed with a little olive oil and parsley spread on toast. Valnet claims to use garlic in preparations to fight intestinal parasites and tapeworm; to dis-

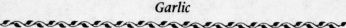

infect sores, wounds, and ulcers; and to treat corns and warts. Garlic oil withdraws the venom from wasp stings and insect bites of all sorts. In soups or eaten raw, garlic cloves provide an excellent remedy for winter respiratory infections and common colds. Even more eye-opening is the fact that a number of clinical studies have illustrated that garlic lowers cholesterol and blood pressure.

As its vigorous aroma might suggest, garlic stimulates and vitalizes. This may explain why a renowned artist, when asked if he felt offended by the smell of garlic on a person's breath, replied, "No, I feel envious!" However, some people avoid garlic because they do not like the way it lingers on the breath. But this should not be a deterrent. There are two other herbs whose high chlorophyll content will neutralize garlic rather easily. After eating garlic, if one chews on a little sweet basil or parsley, "garlic breath" instantly dissipates! Furthermore, there are now several commercially packaged garlic capsules, ranging from 30 to 100 percent garlic in content, that are encased to prevent afterodor. In any case, garlic should be avoided by nursing mothers because its flavor is so strong that it spoils her milk and produces colic in the infant.

The principal constituent of garlic is the volatile oil sulphuretted glucoside.

- Insures fitness and feeling of well-being.
- Enhances immunity to infections.
- Fights intestinal parasites.
- Disinfects wounds and sores.
- Remedy for colds.
- Lowers blood pressure and cholesterol.

Geranium

Pelargonium Odorantissimum (Geraniaceae)

The scented geranium originated in Algeria, Reunion Island off the coast of Africa, Madagascar, and Guinea. As a result of hybridizing, there are now over seven hundred species in the geranium family. These showy plants have one energetic flowering a year and tolerate a blazing summer sun fairly well. They generally grow to be about two feet tall. In many climates, geraniums are popular potted plants, treated as annuals, but they do grow wild in some hedgerows and wooded areas.

The geranium is a chameleonlike plant; if one takes a leaf sample from a number of different varieties one will encounter an array of different fragrances—from rose to lemon to ginger, strawberry, peppermint, camphor, and so forth. For this reason, geranium leaves are often used in potpourri and sachets. The fruitier varieties are used in teas, jams, and as an unusual flavoring in desserts.

Almost as different as its various fragrances are the uses to which it has been put. The ancients believed that the geranium had the power to mend fractures and eliminate cancers. Geraniums were brought from Africa back to the courts of Europe by botanists seeking exotic plants for the royal gardens. And according to the "language of flowers" developed by bored but imaginative Victorian ladies, a sprig of lemon geranium left in an unannounced guest's quarters was a subtle hint that he or she should have written ahead.

Geranium oil, which is clear to pale green, is also multifarious in aromatherapy. It is used in water as a mouthwash to treat tonsillitis and inflammations of the mouth, throat, and tongue. Reputedly, geranium oil makes an excellent treatment for burns and, in general, will reduce inflammations. Furthermore, it is a mild painkiller and is especially helpful when one is suffering from pain that originates more from nerves than a physical trauma. The essence makes a very refreshing bath oil because, like rosemary and basil, it stimulates the adrenal cortex, which produces steroids, thereby stabilizing the nervous system and alleviating stress. Its terpene content (usually found in resins) makes it a powerful mosquito repellant. Finally, geranium oil makes a superb contribution to skin care; it refreshes, invigorates, and clears the skin, combating oily, congested complexions or inflammations.

Geranium essence blends easily with basil, rose, and citrus oils.

- Treats inflammations, especially in the mouth.
- Mild painkiller.
- Alleviates stress and stabilizes the nervous system.
- Clears the skin and reduces skin infections.

Hyssop

Hyssopus Officinalis (Labiatae)

Hyssop, native to southern Europe, is a shrubby, squat evergreen with small blue flowers and tiny pointed leaves. It grows modestly in rocky, dry, out-of-the-way places. In the first English book about English plants, William Turner claimed that the elusive scent of hyssop could "driveth away the Winde that is in the ears."

Hyssop has been valued at intervals all around the globe. The herb derived its name from the ancient Hebrews, who saw it as a sacred plant. They named it *ezob*, which has been transliterated to "hyssop." Hippocrates used it to treat pleurisy. It was cultivated in England and brought to the New World by settlers to make teas and medicinal "cigarettes."

The essential oil of hyssop is pale yellow and very expensive. It is used as an ingredient in some of the most sophisticated perfumes and pricey liqueurs. Hyssop is a primary ingredient in the famous herbal elixir of Grand-Chartreuse. The oil is volatile, thus its reputation for clearing and energizing mental faculties.

For centuries, it has been claimed that hyssop tea, made from the flowers, relieves catarrh. Because of its expecto-

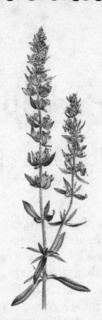

Hyssop (*Hyssopus officinalis*)

rant, tonic, antiseptic, and antispasmodic properties, hyssop essence has also been found to modify expectoration, alleviate difficulty in breathing, and negate chronic coughs.

Hyssop contains ketones, thus, in very high doses it may induce epileptic fits in those predisposed to them. It is, according to the French doctor Caujolle, the only herb capable of doing so. Because of its potential toxicity, hyssop oil should be avoided during pregnancy.

- Stimulates and clears the respiratory system.
- Antiseptic, tonic.
- Should not be used during pregnancy.

Jasmine

Jasminum Officinale and *J. Grandiflorum (Jasminaceae)*

Jasmine is a gracefully arching shrub belonging to the olive family. It grows four to eight feet high. It is evergreen in warmer climates with bright green to dark glossy green foliage. Its most striking characteristic, however, is the intoxicatingly fragrant flowers of yellow, white, or red. This genus produces some of the most fragrant flowers in the world. This is probably one reason why it has been cultivated all over: Algeria, China, Egypt, France, Italy, Morocco, Turkey, and the United States. The most coveted oil comes from the variety cultivated in France, while the Chinese variety is primarily used for scented teas.

The name "jasmine" comes from an Arabic word, *yasmin*, meaning "king." Jasmine was thus named because it was considered to be the king of aromas. And there are many who would agree. Although jasmine does not boast as impressive a list of healing properties as some plant essences, most people find the fragrance irresistible and lavishly erotic.

As a sedative and antidepressant, jasmine essence is most effective against psychological ills such as chronic listlessness, apathy, or melancholy. It induces a sense of euphoria, self-possession, and hopefulness. The primary action is warming and expansive, therefore, it is useful against all the manifestations of nervous disability.

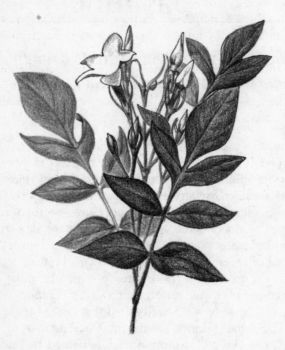

Jasmine (*Jasminum officinale*)

Like the essence of rose, jasmine has a potent remedial impact on the female reproductive system. It relieves menstrual cramps and back pain, reduces labor pains, and encourages the flow of milk. In addition, because it is extremely relaxing and the fragrance is so highly sensual, jasmine combats frigidity and impotence in either sex. It makes an exquisite but extravagant massage oil.

Essence of jasmine is very expensive, thus it is only used in the costliest perfumes. Although perfume is the principal cosmetic application for this oil, used in moderation, jasmine benefits hot, dry skin, especially in the case of itching or redness. It is sometimes used in hair conditioners for treating dry scalps. The oil itself is quite aesthetically pleasing with its sweet, exuberant bouquet and beautiful, deep chestnut color.

- Sedative.
- Antidepressant, induces euphoria and hopefulness.
- Remedies frigidity and impotence.
- Moisturizer, heals skin problems.

Juniper

Juniperus Communis (Coniferae)

The juniper is a small hardwood evergreen shrub native to central and southern Europe, Sweden, Canada, and North America. It thrives in full sun. It has needlelike foliage that ranges from dark green to steel-blue. Some varieties have prominent, colorful fruit.

Cato the Elder, of ancient Rome, was the first to write about the antiseptic and diuretic properties of juniper. But long before, in Tibet, it was burned as incense in religious ceremonies. In the New Testament, it is reported that juniper branches provided protection for Mary and the baby Jesus as they fled from King Herod. Medieval herbalists used it to ward off evil spirits and disinfect the air when plagues and other contagious diseases were running rampant. Until recently, some French and Yugoslavian hospitals burned juniper twigs (often with rosemary leaves) to purify the air and refresh sickrooms.

"Cade oil" is extracted from the trunks of mature juniper trees; it is used for dermatosis and toothaches. But the more therapeutic oil is obtained from the dark, currantlike berries (which are also used to make gin). The oil is a pale yellowish green color with a surprisingly pleasant fragrance, surprising because it is reminiscent of turpentine. As a bath oil, it is both relaxing and stimulating, like pine and cypress oils.

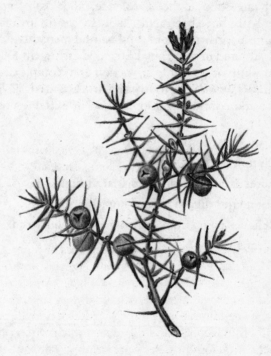

Juniper (*Juniperus communis*)

Botanically, juniper is closely related to cypress. While it is less potent than cypress as an antispasmodic and astringent, it is more effective as a diuretic. It is a classic cure for urinary tract infections.

Juniper essence is exceptionally versatile considering its exceedingly low toxicity. In general, the berries stimulate secretions and promote purification. Juniper is indicated for sluggish digestion, colic, flatulence, and loss of appetite. Juniper baths have been remarkably successful in combating rheumatism, arthritis, gout, and painful menstruation. Juniper oil, diluted in water, makes a good astringent for toning normal skin or treating an acne-beset complexion. Although it is never wise to overuse any essential oil, juniper produces no contraindications, even in extreme dosages.

- Antiseptic, tonic.
- Diuretic.
- Cures infections of the urinary tract.
- Stimulates digestion and improves appetite.
- Relieves pains from arthritis and rheumatism.
- Cleans skin.

Lavender

Lavandula Officinalis (Labiatae)

Lavender is a sweet-scented herb in the mint family that produces spikes of pale purple flowers. It is a shrubby plant indigenous to mountainous regions of Europe. The fundamental motivation for cultivating this plant is for the distillation of its oil. As it is one of the most commercially popular essences, it is known as the "universal oil." Together England, France, Yugoslavia, Tasmania, and Bulgaria produce most of the world's lavender oil. The French variety is the oldest and most highly prized.

For centuries, the clean, penetrating scent of lavender oil has been used to alleviate tension headaches and, according to the seventeenth-century English herbalist Nicholas Culpeper, falling sickness or giddiness of the brain. Lavender was the favorite bath oil of the Romans, from whom the herb gets its name: The Latin word *lavare* means "to wash."

Lavender, with its unique clean, fresh, floral scent, is the chief ingredient in most sachets, potpourri, and many toilet waters. It is the touch of mystery in the famous Herbes de Provence. Dried lavender is also used to keep linen fresh and to keep away moths.

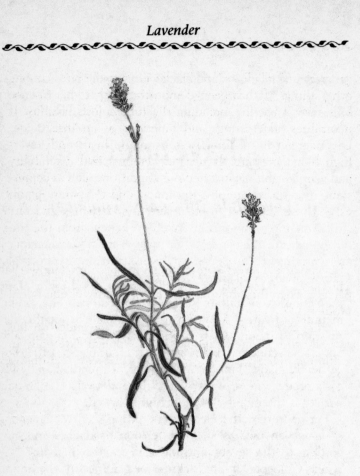

Lavender (*Lavandula officinalis*)

Aromatherapists and herbalists claim that lavender is among the most useful and versatile essences. In 1938, Gattefosse published an article in which he related discoveries of the significant power of lavender essence to heal gangrene, facial ulcers, and black widow spider bites, among other things. It has been demonstrated that this essence kills sever̠l bacilli, including the tuberculosis bacillus. It neutralizes adder stings and functions as an insecticide. Lavender oil has a tonic action on the heart and lowers high blood pressure. It negates cerebrospinal excitability and is invaluable against nervous conditions such as depression, hysteria, migraines, insomnia, and temporary paralysis. Those suffering from violent mood swings and any strong mental symptoms are likely to benefit from the stabilizing effects of lavender. The antispasmodic, stomachic, and carminative properties of lavender make it effectual against a variety of digestive or respiratory problems, especially when the ailments are related to stress or emotional problems.

Aside from being a favorite perfume, lavender oil has several other cosmetic applications. Applied externally in a diluted solution, the oil rejuvenates oily skin, eliminates acne and eczema, and subdues scars.

- Relieves headaches.
- Remedies nervous conditions and stress.
- Lowers high blood pressure.
- Insect repellant.
- Antiseptic and tonic.

Lemon

Citrus Limonum (Rutaceae)

The lemon tree is a small, spiny, semitropical evergreen tree of the rue family. Botanists believe that the lemon tree originated in India. It grows heartily in southern Europe, especially Spain and Portugal. Rich in vitamin C, the fruit and the essence have numerous medicinal and cosmetic applications.

In Spain, where citrus trees grow exuberantly, lemon essence is used systematically to treat countless ills and with evident success. The essence is obtained from the fruit's rind. Green fruit yields more essence than ripe fruit. Lemon juice, on the other hand, is most easily obtained if the ripe fruit is soaked in warm water for five minutes before squeezing.

Mediterranean cuisine's abundant use of lemon is more than a matter of taste. Lemon juice is both a disinfectant and a preservative. Lack of refrigeration in peasant communities prompted the discovery. In many circumstances, lemon juice may be used to disinfect doubtful drinking water or meat.

Lemons have numerous practical, non-health-related uses. Half a lemon rubbed in rock salt can be used to remove tarnish from brasswork. A slice of lemon rinsed in warm water will polish silver. Lemon and a hot iron will remove rust stains from white linen. Fingers stained with ink or other juices can be cleaned with lemon juice. In addition, dried lemon rind hanging in a closet will repel moths, while rotten lemons, placed strategically in a garden, will repel ants.

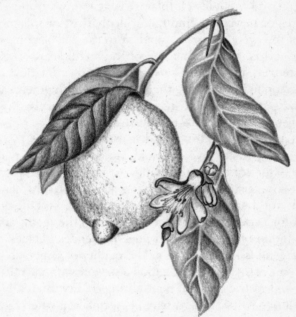

Lemon (*Citrus limonum*)

Although the essence is used by aromatherapists in medicinal draughts, even the relatively inexperienced can aptly use lemon juice against a variety of ailments. Drops of juice applied to the nostrils several times daily clear head colds and sinus trouble. A saturated cotton pad held against

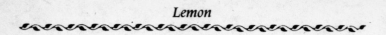

the nose will stop a nosebleed. Applied to cuts or wounds, the juice acts as an antiseptic and promotes scar development. Gargling with warm water and lemon juice soothes tonsillitis, sore throats, and mouth sores. Compresses of lemon juice applied to the forehead eliminate migraines. Rubbed into the skin, lemon juice protects the body against the cold and mollifies chilblains. A few drops of juice in the eyes of newborns eliminates blepharitis, or inflammation of the eyelids. Finally, applied to the ear, lemon juice reduces otitis, or inflammation of the middle ear.

Moreover, the lemon serves numerous cosmetic functions. Applied externally, the rind mixed with vinegar will eliminate warts. Lemon juice softens brittle nails. As an astringent, the juice makes an excellent skin toner for an oily complexion, and it is said to banish wrinkles. Mixed with equal parts of glycerine and eau de cologne, it makes a lotion for softening the hands. It will also soften and soothe sore feet if rubbed on after a warm footbath. Lemon juice is antidotal to insect bites. And finally, because of its bleaching action, lemon juice can whiten the teeth, and a facial lotion of slightly salted juice moderates freckles.

Everyone is aware of the acidic quality of lemon, but it may come as a surprise that lemon also works as an alkalizing agent and gastric antacid, neutralizing acidity internally. A hyperactive gastric system may be normalized when lemon juice is added to the diet.

- Relieves head colds and sinus trouble.
- Antiseptic, astringent, tonic.
- Promotes scar development.
- Stimulates the digestive system.

Marjoram

Origanum Marjorana (Labiatea)

Marjoram is indigenous to the Mediterranean coast, Persia, Hungary, and Yugoslavia. It produces pink and white flowers in the summer. Although it is in the mint family, the flavor of its leaves is closer to that of oregano (also in the mint family). Marjoram has a warm, pungently sweet fragrance and has long been a popular culinary herb.

Aside from its usefulness in seasoning meats, vegetables, and soups, various civilizations have recognized the medicinal value of marjoram. The Greeks used it to treat dropsy, narcotic poisoning, and convulsions. They used it in cosmetic products such as perfumes and bath oils.

Marjoram is chiefly antispasmodic and sedative. It has been used to remedy insomnia, migraines, anxiety, mental instability, digestive and respiratory spasms, and high blood pressure. Applied externally as part of a massage, marjoram oil can soothe tense or strained muscles, sprains, and rheumatism. It has a warming influence on the autonomic nervous system and induces dilation of the blood vessels. Because it both relaxes and expands, many professional singers have used an infusion of marjoram sweetened with honey as a natural preservative for their instruments: their throat and vocal cords!

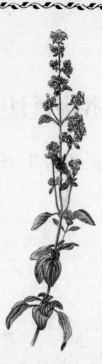

Marjoram (*Origanum marjorana*)

Marjoram oil blends quite well with bergamot and lavender.

- Antispasmodic and sedative.
- Relieves mental instability.
- Remedies insomnia, migraine, anxiety.
- Soothes muscle strains.
- Lowers high blood pressure.
- Calms digestive and respiratory spasms.

Myrrh

Commiphora Myrrha (Burseraceae)

Myrrh is a gum resin, fragrant but bitter tasting. The myrrh bush grows in the deserts of Arabia and East Africa. The branches are gnarled and hard; when they are wounded or split the resin naturally seeps out. At first it has a yellowish hue, then it dries into a reddish brown color. The essence likewise is a lovely reddish mahogany color. Myrrh has a smoky aroma, not especially sweet, but exotic and inviting.

Along with frankincense, myrrh was the most popular essence of the ancient world. It has been in use for over three thousand years in incense, perfumes, and other beauty and health-care treatments. On the battlefield, the Greeks used myrrh to treat wounds and reduce inflammations. In Egypt, myrrh was burned daily at high noon as part of a sun-worshiping ceremony. It was also employed in the Egyptian embalming process. Because of its preserving property, the Egyptians discovered that myrrh makes a splendid cosmetic. A recipe for a facial mask using myrrh was found on the Ebers papyrus dating from the eighteenth Egyptian dynasty (ca. 1580 B.C.)

Medicinally, myrrh is antiinflammatory and antiseptic. It is a healing stimulant, effective against indolent wounds and stomach ulcers. A mouthwash made out of half a teaspoon of myrrh, a dash of cayenne pepper, and three ounces of water medicates gum infections and eliminates bad breath. Its chief action is expectorant, thus myrrh is effective against coughs, bronchitis, and instances of mucus buildup. However, myrrh also stimulates digestion, stirring gastric juices and eliminating flatulence.

- Preservative.
- Antiseptic and antiinflammatory agent.
- Expectorant.
- Reduces mucus buildup.
- Stimulates the digestive process.
- Heals infected wounds.

Onion

Allium Cepa (Liliaceae)

The onion, like garlic, is a member of the lily family. The
bulb, which is edible, has a strong, sharp taste. Although
the essence of onion is not commonly used because it is
rather acrid, the intact onion, with its powerful yet slightly
sweet aroma, is very effective in treating illnesses.

Dioscorides, a Greek doctor of the first century A.D.,
praised the onion's capacity to fight infection and its tonic
and diuretic properties. Today, knowledge of the onion's
constituents—which include iron, sulfur, silica, potassium
salts, iodine, phosphates, and nitrates—allows medics to
understand the effects detected by the pioneers of aromatherapy. In the 1970s, Professor Kharchenko, the chair of
the department of pharmacology at a Soviet medical insti-
tute, completed a ten-year study of the onion. He found
that the onion is rich in vitamins C and B, carotene, and
has antibiotic, digestive, and cardiotonic properties.

Most people appreciate the culinary value of the onion.
However, it also boasts an extraordinary number of healing
properties. Onions have been used to administer to physical
and mental fatigue, the retention of liquids, obesity, gallstones, diabetes, genitourinary infections, respiratory ail-

ments, glandular imbalance, impotence, and intestinal parasites. Applied externally, an onion can treat insect bites and wasp stings, while cut onions repel mosquitoes. Onion soup is said to cure flatulence, indigestion, and hangovers. Because of its gluconin, the onion has been valuable in cases of diabetes.

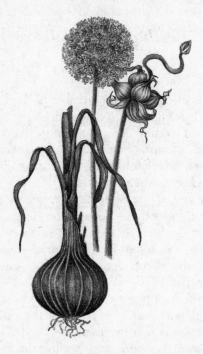

Onion (*Allium cepa*)

Proponents of natural medicine have recorded numerous simple remedies involving the onion. A poultice of raw onions applied to the forehead for migraines and to the abdomen for retention of urine has proven effective. Onion juice applied to chapped lips, chafed skin, or chilblains has curative results. The thin membrane found between each layer of an onion can be used as an antiseptic for wounds, burns, and cuts. Chopped onions boiled in a few cups of water will cure diarrhea. Finally, the aroma from a slice of onion held close to the nose will settle the nerves and ward off hysteria.

- Fights infections.
- Diuretic.
- Combats physical and mental fatigue.
- Treats insect bites and stings.
- Balances the glandular system.
- Cures digestive ailments.

Orange Blossom (Neroli)

Citrus Aurantium (Rutaceae)

The tree from which neroli oil is extracted is known as the bitter orange tree or the Seville orange. It originated in China but now grows in Mediterranean areas, California, Mexico, South America, and near the Indian Ocean.

It seems that Portuguese sailors returning from the East Indies brought orange trees to Europe. These trees instantly found popularity in the courts and became featured specimens in formal gardens.

The essence is obtained through distillation of the flowers. It is pale yellow in color. Although the taste of the oil is bitter, the aroma is sweet, full-bodied, and luscious. It blends well with a number of other oils, providing a solid backbone to floral perfume combinations. Neroli oil, blended with lavender, rosemary, lemon, and bergamot oils, creates eau de cologne.

Neroli's action is chiefly sedative, even slightly hypnotic, so it has proven effective against insomnia, anxiety attacks, general tension, and stress-related illnesses. This oil also settles heart palpitations and counters shock.

Neroli is further recommended as a natural deodorant. Because it is extremely mild, it may be applied directly to the skin or it may be used in a bath, where it will serve to relax mind and body as well as rehabilitate and scent blemished skin. Because the oil is so mild it is appropriate for calming agitated or colicky infants.

- Soothes sensitive skin.
- Relieves tension and stress-related illness.
- Sedative.
- Natural deodorant.

Patchouli

Pogostemon Patchouli (Labiatae)

Patchouli is a robust East Indian mint that grows to three or four feet in height. The leaves of the plant are fairly large and egg-shaped; the flowers are a pale lavender color. A heavy, dark brown oil with an evocative, exotic fragrance is derived from the leaves. The oil has the unique property of aging well, like a good vintage wine. And like wines, patchouli has been compared by aromatherapists to any number of things: musty clothes, ancient attics, and vigorous goats! Despite the connotations suggested by these comparisons, all seem to agree that the scent has an earthy appeal, and the oil is widely used in the manufacture of soaps and perfumes. However, all agree that the taste is notably sour and unpleasant.

Patchouli and its oil were brought to England by importers in the late nineteenth century. The fragrant scent was used to attract buyers to products from India. Long before this, in India, the oil was being used to scent sachets, potpourris, and linen. When sprinkled on clothing, it deters moths. The scent of patchouli, blended with camphor, gives Indian ink its characteristic aroma.

The most interesting feature of patchouli is its dualistic constitution. In small doses it acts as a stimulant, while in large doses it has a sedative effect—causing loss of appetite and sleepiness. This dual nature makes patchouli an especially potent aphrodisiac. Furthermore, patchouli oil is a mild astringent, but it has the agreeable characteristic of constricting only where there is inordinate looseness. It inhibits where there is excessive flow—of mucus, skin oil, menstrual blood, water, or diarrhea; it will not impede natural flow. Patchouli is said to have an analogous impact on the mind, focusing one's thoughts when there is an absence of clarity or concentration and easing anxiety.

- In small doses: stimulant.
- In large doses: sedative.
- Mild astringent.
- Reduces excessive flow of body fluids.
- Improves ability to concentrate and focus.

Peppermint

Mentha Piperita (Labiatae)

There are many kinds of mints grown throughout the world. Mint will grow almost anywhere and tends to be hardy to the point of invasiveness. In fact, the only problem with mint is that its exuberance can be difficult to control. However, this particular mint is grown widely in America, England, Italy, and France. For the indifferent gardener it is, of course, a dream come true!

The generic name for this aromatic group, *Mentha*, comes from Greek mythology. Menthe was a lovely nymph with whom Hades, ruler of the underworld, fell in love. Hades' wife, Persephone, learned of this infatuation and decided to seek revenge. Persephone pursued Menthe and then trampled her into the ground. Later, Hades took pity on Menthe and transformed the nymph into the vigorous plant we now so readily consume.

Peppermint has endured for quite a long time. The Pharisees of Egypt paid their tithes with parcels of mint, cumin, and anise. The Romans, who brought the herb to Britain, were very fond of mint; Pliny writes that the Romans as well as the Greeks crowned themselves with wreaths of peppermint on feast days. Mint was valued in the cloistered gardens of early monasteries, and numerous references to it can be found in the texts left by medieval herbalists. In America, mint was already growing wild before settlers arrived, bringing more varieties along with them. Some North American Indians used peppermint leaves to treat pneumonia. Today, in traditional Texas households, a bundle

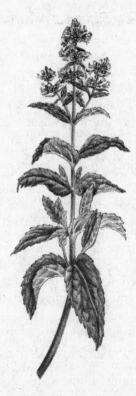

Peppermint (*Mentha piperita*)

of mint in a vase by the doorway is said to sweeten a guest's arrival; in the Middle East, hot mint tea is a symbol of salutation to the wayfarer or new visitor.

Peppermint is still put to many uses. Its oil as well as the dried and fresh leaves are employed imaginatively in numerous cuisines. Medicines, toothpastes, and mouthwashes are scented with mint. Both the leaves and the essence of peppermint are used in aromatherapy.

The essence is procured from the leaves and flowering tops through steam distillation. The oil is clear and it has a sharp, clean, refreshing smell familiar to almost everyone. The taste is simultaneously bitter, sweet, and sour. America is responsible for producing the most oil, but the European oils are regarded as qualitatively superior.

Peppermint is one of the most versatile essences. Menthol is the chief constituent of this oil and is responsible for most of its healing properties. Used in inhalations, the expectorant property of peppermint can relieve asthma, bronchitis, and sinus congestion; inflammation; or infection. Its antispasmodic properties have proved useful in some purgatives. Peppermint tea soothes the stomach, stops vomiting, abates flatulence and colic, cures sea and car sickness, and aids with digestion—this last explains the tradition of concluding dinner with a mint. Peppermint essence acts as a stimulant on the nervous system and is a far safer and more reliable remedy than aspirin. Applied externally, it can counter migraines, toothache, fevers, and general aches and pains. An infusion of the essence can inhibit sleep at night, but some use it specifically for this purpose—as a natural, safe alternative to caffeine. Peppermint oil has also been used to treat gallstones, anemia, and scanty menstruation.

Peppermint oil has a healing influence on skin disorders. It has been used to medicate scabies, ringworm, and shingles. It will relieve itching, redness, inflammation, and acne. However, it should be used in moderation, otherwise it may aggravate the condition. Peppermint both cools and warms; it cools overheated skin by constricting the capillaries, and invigorates a pale, sallow complexion. Peppermint oil in a bath will lower body temperature, providing some relief from sunburn or the lethargy one feels on a hot summer day. If one takes it along on camping trips, a few drops in the tent will repel mosquitoes. Having neglected to take this preventative measure, peppermint oil will soothe the itching of most insect bites.

- Antispasmodic.
- Antiseptic.
- Heals skin disorders.
- Relieves pains and aches.
- Expectorant.
- Stimulates the digestive functions.
- Safe alternative to caffeine.

Pine

Pinus Sylestris (Pinaceae)

This particular pine is also known as Scots (or Scotch) pine. It is an evergreen tree that produces hard, woody cones and bundles of two to five needlelike leaves. It grows extensively in cold, upland regions of Russia, Europe, Scandinavia, and North America.

In 1534, Jacques Cartier learned from the American Indians that extracts of pine needles can cure and prevent scurvy, a disease resulting from a deficiency of vitamin C. Pines have long been valued for their wood and resin, from which both turpentine and tar are derived. And although not fully exploited, pine is still used medicinally today.

Several parts of the pine are used in aromatherapy: the buds; the thick, distilled resin; and the oil, which is obtained from the needles through steam distillation. The essence has a fresh, woody, balsamic aroma.

Taken internally, pine oil is a powerful antiseptic of the respiratory, urinary, and hepatic systems. Thus, it is useful in treating all respiratory tract infections, such as bronchitis, pneumonia, asthma, and common colds, as well as urinary infections and gallstones. Pine essence stimulates the adrenal cortex, where a variety of steroids are produced,

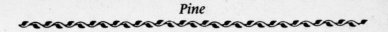

making it effective against impotence. Both the buds and the essence, used in local baths, act as rubefacients, combating rheumatic complaints and gout. They will also alleviate excessive perspiration.

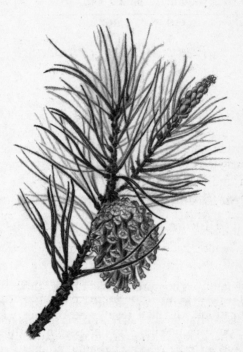

Pine (*Pinus sylestris*)

Used in a diffuser and deeply inhaled, pine oil has a warming, revitalizing, and comforting influence on the psyche. It is a gentle panacea for emotional stress.

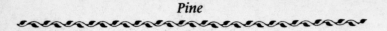

- Antiseptic of the respiratory, urinary, and hepatic systems.
- Relieves emotional stress.
- Effective against impotence.
- Soothes rheumatic pains.
- Reduces excessive perspiration.

Rose

Rosa Damascena—Damask Rose, Rosa Centifolia—Cabbage Rose (Rosaceae)

The rose family is comprised of some two thousand species, including trees, herbs, and shrubs. The rose is a remarkably hearty plant that grows easily in diverse soils and climates all over the globe. However, it does particularly well in temperate and mild zones. Fossil specimens of the rose indicate that some strains have been growing on the North American continent for at least thirty-two million years! In the past few centuries, the adaptability of the rose has been utilized extensively; thousands of varieties have been developed through hybridization. Attar, the essence of rose, is used in many perfumes and toiletries. Rose hips, the fruit

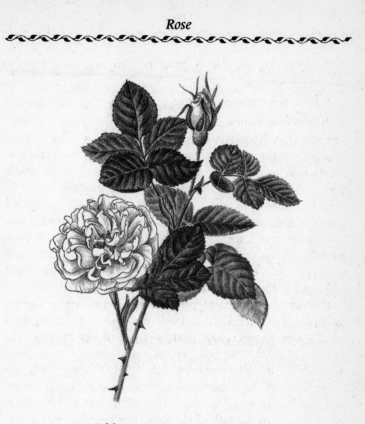

Cabbage Rose (*Rosa centifolia*)

produced by many rose varieties, contain a very high concentration of vitamin C.

For centuries, the rose has occupied a prominent place
in all aspects of human culture: art, literature, medicine,
beautification, and, of course, horticulture. Greek writers
made poetic references to the rose as early as 600 B.C.
Representations of the rose can be seen in Egyptian art and
architecture and on Abyssinian tombs dating from the first
to fifth centuries A.D. This suggests that roses may have

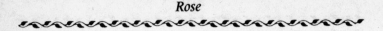

been construed as an especially suitable funeral offering. We know that Cleopatra used roses in ceremonial rites as well as in her elaborate cosmetic rituals. The rose garden of King Midas was one of the wonders of the ancient world. The ancient Romans were largely responsible for widely disseminating the rose; they planted rose and herb gardens everywhere they conquered. Romans used roses in garlands, perfumes, baths, sweets, and hangover remedies.

In Greek and Roman mythology, the rose is associated with the goddess of love: Aphrodite/Venus. Reputedly, the rose originated either as a result of her first tears or as a birthday gift from the other gods when she initially emerged from the sea. There are several myths meant to explain the rose's red color. In one version, Aphrodite was seeking her lost lover, Adonis, and pricked her fingers on a thorny rosebush; her blood then dyed the flowers red. Another story attributes the characteristic color to her mischievous son, Cupid, who supposedly spilled a glass of wine on a virginal shrub. In a different tale, Cupid is also held accountable for the thorns: While bending to smell an especially lovely rose, he was stung by a bee; in his anger, he shot an arrow, missed the bee, but permanently penetrated the rosebush.

On a metaphoric level, these myths help clarify why the rose has long been viewed as an apt symbol of romantic love. Because the rose stimulates virtually all of the five senses, it, like love, can be intoxicating. However, while its blossom appears delicate, it can leave the blind pursuer bleeding if he or she fails to heed the thorns.

Despite the hazards suggested by the above analogy, rose essence is actually the least toxic of all essential oils. In keeping with expectations, the scent is exquisite: agreeable,

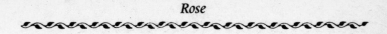

intensely sweet, and robust. Without needing the evidence provided by contemporary aromatherapists, many cultures have recognized that the especially pleasant and potent fragrance acts as an antidepressant as well as an aphrodisiac. But contrary to expectation, rose oil is not red, but a greenish orange color. It may also come as a surprise that rose is among the most antiseptic of the essential oils. Thus, rose essence is an excellent skin tonic, appropriate for sensitive, damaged, or dry complexions, and, applied on the eyes, heals conjunctivitis and inflammation.

Legend has it that rose oil was first discovered during a wedding feast in Persia. A canal, encircling the royal gardens, had been filled with rose water. The sun's heat caused the oil to separate and float to the top. The oil was collected and examined. Recognizing the myriad possibilities inherent in this floral "by-product," the Persians began to produce it for commercial distribution.

Today, the best and most expensive rose oil comes from Bulgaria, where it is extracted from damask roses, so named because they were brought back to Europe by the Crusaders from Damascus. It takes approximately thirty roses to make a single drop of Bulgarian oil—and sixty thousand roses to make an ounce! Large-scale cultivation of the centifolia rose, used extensively in the manufacture of perfumes, takes place in southern France.

All medieval herbalists from whom we have retained records cite the healing properties of the rose. They all stress its cathartic and soothing characteristics. Proponents of herbal medicine have long been aware of the interesting connection between the distinctly feminine fragrance and shape of the rose and its usefulness in regulating "feminine" health problems. Rose oil can be used to regulate the men-

133

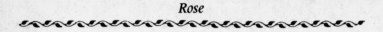

strual cycle and treat all genitourinary tract disorders. Rose hip tea is one of the best and safest remedies for menstrual cramps.

The rose has been used in ministering to other systemic problems as well. It has a purging action on the vascular and digestive systems. As a vascular stimulant, rose tones the capillaries, improves circulation, cleanses the blood, and regulates the heart and spleen. In cleansing the digestive system, it is useful for eliminating excess bile, strengthening the stomach, and treating constipation, nausea, and vomiting. The triple action of rose oil on the nervous, vascular, and digestive systems makes it effective in medicating the physical manifestations of stress such as stomach ulcers, heart disease, and anxiety attacks.

The rose has been used to scent a multitude of products: candles, honey, vinegar, wine, throat lozenges, snuff, gourmet sauces, and, of course, potpourri. In terms of cosmetics, rose-scented commodities—perfumes, soaps, lotions, and bath salts—remain the most popular worldwide. The most expensive perfume made, Joy, is a splash of jasmine oil and lots of roses.

- Strong antiseptic.
- Tonic, especially for sensitive skin.
- Soothes.
- Regulates female conditions and cycles.
- Treats genitourinary problems.
- Purging agent.
- Regulates the digestive system.

Rosemary

Rosmarinus Officinalis (Labiatae)

Rosemary is an intensely fragrant evergreen herb of the mint family. Its scientific name means "dew of the sea" because of its preference for warm, sea-sprayed locations. It is native to the Mediterranean, Yugoslavia, Guatemala, and Costa Rica. However, this especially renowned herb is grown and sold all over the world. The shrub grows up to six feet in height and produces intermittent clusters of small, powder blue flowers and richly resinous foliage that is soft to the touch. The small, spiky leaves are silvery gray underneath and dark green on top. They are so aromatic that one need only brush a spray through a hand to release a scent that will linger for quite a while. For this reason, rosemary is considered a symbol of remembrance.

In the Western world, rosemary is probably the most popular herb and the herb with the most involved legacy. Although it is much acclaimed as a culinary herb, rosemary has been put to many other uses. Early Greek philosophers wore garlands of rosemary to stimulate the brain and promote memory retention. Because of its association with memory, it has long been used in wedding bouquets and

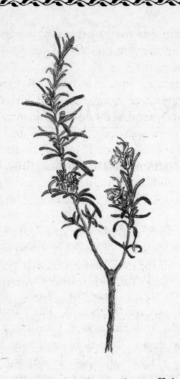

Rosemary (*Rosmarinus officinalis*)

wreaths as a symbol for fidelity and in funereal wreaths as
a pledge to remember the departed. Pliny insisted that the
herb was good for jaundice, failing eyesight, and healing
wounds; all of these claims were seconded by Nicholas Culpeper in the seventeenth century. In the sixth century,
Charlemagne declared that this herb should be grown in
all of the imperial gardens. Up until the 1950s, rosemary

sprays were still being burned in the sickrooms of hospitals as a means for purging the air of evil spirits—literally as well as symbolically.

Rosemary fragrance, which is fiery, invigorating, and camphoreous, is effective against mental fatigue, memory loss, disorientation, and melancholy. In aromatherapy, the leaves and flower tops are used in infusions and the essence is derived from the flower tops through steam distillation. However, simply rubbing one's hands against branches of the growing plant and then inhaling the scent can be mildly rehabilitating, especially against headaches and emotional fatigue.

The oil is clear with a sharp but nonbitter taste. A little of the oil mixed with some olive oil makes a sensuous and effective massage oil for muscular rheumatic pains. The oil in a bath is revitalizing. Taken internally, rosemary relieves disturbances of the liver, painful digestion, gastric pains, and colitis. This essence has a pronounced remedial effect on the nervous system, correcting motor impairments, migraines, tension headaches, and vertigo; in excessive quantities, rosemary essence can induce epilepsy. Rosemary essence is used as a tonic for nervous cardiac conditions, such as palpitations, and it will normalize both high cholesterol and low blood pressure. Being a mild stimulant, it is good for countering apathy, lethargy, and general debility.

Rosemary oil has several cosmetic properties. In the fourteenth century, Queen Elizabeth of Hungary used rosemary water as a facial wash and rejuvenating lotion. It heals dry skin, reduces hair loss, and cures dandruff, while adding body and shine to hair and invigorating a pasty complexion. It is a powerful natural deodorant and air freshener.

Rosemary is a significant component of eau de cologne, and because of the healing action rosemary essence has on the nervous system, a little eau de cologne applied to the temples will help relieve minor, nagging headaches.

- Fights mental fatigue.
- Stimulates memory.
- Calms rheumatic pains.
- Revitalizes.
- Relieves digestive pains.
- A natural deodorant and air freshener.

Sage

Salvia Officinalis (Labiatae)

Sage is a very large genus of the mint family, and "garden sage" is the most common. This hardy shrub usually keeps its leaves during the winter, although in some regions it has difficulty making it through harsh summers. It is grown throughout the world for its aromatic leaves. The leaves are broad, slightly wrinkled, and gray in color. Sage is a significant culinary herb: The English use it to season cheese; the Russians, holiday goose; and Americans, Thanksgiving turkey and dressing. However, it has been a popular home remedy for ages.

The Latin name *salvere*, from which we get "salvia," means "to be saved." In fact, sage has a long history as a medicinal plant. While the Romans viewed it as sacred, sage was also the most celebrated herbal medicine in the Middle Ages, used for everything from relieving headaches to bestowing wisdom. Extant receipts from seventeenth-century medics demonstrate that sage was then grown in America for medicinal purposes Several cultures have viewed sage as the plant of eternal youth.

The leaves, flowers, and essence are all used in aromatherapy. The essence is clear with a pleasant, floral scent. One reason why it is such an effective curative is that it is especially potent; large doses can be toxic to the nervous system.

Sage has the following properties: It is tonic, antiseptic, hypertensive, and antispasmodic. It has a restorative effect on the whole body, especially the nervous, digestive, and pulmonary systems. It has been used to treat sluggish digestion, asthma, low blood pressure, and nervous afflictions of all kinds. It is good for cleaning the teeth and preventing gingivitis, or gum disease. As a gargle or mouthwash sage infusions can treat thrush, mouth ulcers, and inflammations. Dried sage leaves are burned as a room deodorizer and disinfectant. One can apply a poultice of crushed leaves to wasp stings or insect bites. Dr. Jean Valnet claims that regular infusions of sage essence one month before delivery will ease labor pains during childbirth. Likewise, sage has long been recognized as an effective means for regulating the menstrual cycle. Only recently, scientists discovered an explanation for this: Sage contains estrogen, the hormone that encourages menstruation in female mammals.

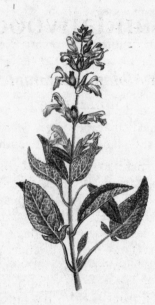

Sage (*Salvia officinalis*)

- Tonic, antiseptic.
- Restores the nervous, digestive, and pulmonary systems.
- Regulates the menstrual cycle.
- Prevents gum disease.
- Deodorizes and disinfects.

Sandalwood

Santalum Album, Santalum Spicatum
(Santalaceae)

Sandalwood is the hard, close-grained, light-colored, sweet-smelling heartwood of an evergreen tree found in the East Indies, parts of China, and Australia. *Santalum album* is the white sandalwood of Asia; *Santalum spicatum* is found in Australia. The trees grow to a height of twenty to thirty feet and produce yellow, red, or lavender-pink flowers.

Sandalwood has been used since antiquity as incense and in cosmetics. It is mentioned in the oldest extant Vedic manuscript, which dates back to the fifth century B.C. In ancient India and Egypt, it was widely used as incense, perfume, and sacred unguent for anointing rulers and high priests. In the East, many valuable pieces of furniture and ornaments for temples were made out of sandalwood because of its pleasant scent and capacity for warding off insects. It remains the most popular fragrance in India today.

Now the trees are reserved for the distillation of essence. The oil is rich and gloppy, pale yellow-green in color, and tastes decidedly bitter. Of all the essences, sandalwood is probably the most valued in perfumery, in its pure form and as a fixative in expensive perfumes. The fragrance is woody, sweet, reminiscent of rose, evocative of the Orient, and for many an aphrodisiac.

Sandalwood has notable antiseptic properties, particularly for treating infections of the genitourinary tract. It has a notable effect on the mucous membranes of the pulmonary as well as the genitourinary system. Its expectorant and antispasmodic properties make it useful for sore throats, chronic coughs, bronchitis, and catarrh. Inhalations of its soothing aroma combat depression and anxiety. However, the heaviness of the oil makes it more sedative than exhilarating.

Sandalwood oil, in cosmetic products or alone, is great for the skin. It is a gentle astringent, alleviating itching, redness, inflammation, and it works as an antiseptic for acne.

- Gentle astringent and antiseptic.
- Treats genitourinary infections.
- Expectorant and antispasmodic.
- Combats depression and anxiety.
- Mild sedative.

Savory

Satureia Montana (Labiatae)

Savory is an evergreen perennial herb with pungent-flavored small leaves and pale lilac flowers. It is a member of the mint family and is native to southern Europe. The species used in aromatherapy is commonly known as winter savory because of its winter hardiness. It has long been used as a culinary herb, especially for masking meat past its prime and energizing anemic vegetables. It is a favorite for seasoning beans and poultry. The flavor of the leaves is slightly rough and peppery.

Many medieval herbalists recommended savory liqueurs to promote digestion, treat mouth and throat ulcers, and relieve toothaches. A recent study conducted by the pharmacological faculty at Montpelier in France demonstrated the impressive antifungal and antibacterial powers of savory essence, so perhaps the older aromatherapists weren't off target.

The essence is obtained through distillation of the flowering tops. This essence is chiefly a digestive and mental stimulant and has been used effectively to treat painful digestion, flatulence, diarrhea, gastric pains with nervous origins, and mental and sexual debility.

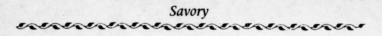

- Antifungal and antibacterial.
- Stimulates digestion and mental powers.

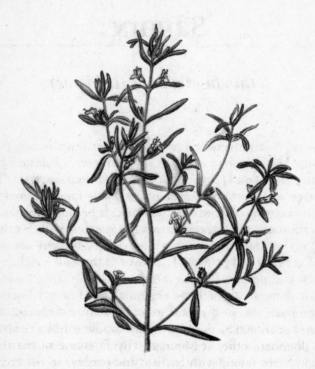

Savory (*Satureia montana*)

Thyme

Thymus Vulgaris (Labiatae)

Thyme is another shrubby herb in the mint family. It is
fairly low-growing, with white, pink, or red flowers and
aromatic leaves. Thyme grows wild on the moors of England
and Scotland. There are something like four hundred varieties of thyme. The count is inexact because thymes are
prolific cross-pollinators; new hybrids emerge all the time.
There are two general categories: upright and creeping
varieties.

The upright species are best for cooking. And thyme is
used profusely in cuisines around the world. It has an es-
pecial affinity with stews, leafy vegetables, legumes, and
fish, but should be used sparingly because it has a tendency
to dominate other seasonings. Thyme is one of the three
main herbs (along with bay leaf and parsley) in the French
bouquet garni.

The name of this herb comes from the Greek *thymon*,
meaning "to offer sacrifice." Its sweet fragrance was thought
to be as pleasing to gods as to mortals, so it was burned as
incense in sacred temples. Furthermore, the ancients believed that our souls inhabited thyme blossoms; thus, a

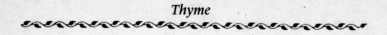

thyme branch bestowed upon the dead was thought to insure safe passage to the underworld.

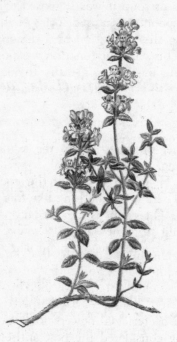

Thyme (*Thymus vulgaris*)

Thyme was very popular in medieval Europe. It was used to make cough syrups, and the Spanish used it to preserve their precious olives. It was brought to America by the earliest settlers. The colonists mixed it with lard to make it more palatable. We now know that thyme has an antioxidant property, which explains the preservative power detected by our predecessors.

Thyme also came to be seen as a symbol of courage. Infused in beer or soup it was supposed to cure shyness. The French Republicans carried sprigs of thyme to secret meetings during the revolution as a designation of their commitment. This symbolic function was not too outlandish, as aromatherapists now identify thyme as a notable physical and mental stimulant, said to sharpen the wits and disperse nervous debility.

In harnessing its diverse therapeutic properties, thyme is used in two forms: infusions made from the leaves and flowering tops, and the essential oil derived from the flowering tops by steam distillation. Both the leaves and the plant essence, called thymol, have a markedly pleasant odor and flavor.

Most of the famous "physicians" of antiquity, such as Dioscorides, Hippocrates, Pliny, and Virgil, employed thyme as a significant healing tool. Contemporary aromatherapists, homeopaths, and herbologists are continuing the legacy. The essence is frequently used in pharmaceutical preparations as well. It has been established that the essence of thyme has a bactericidal power more potent than that of phenol, long considered the best antiseptic available. Thyme is said to provide one of the best remedies for all illnesses resulting from chills, including stubborn head colds. Its antispasmodic and expectorant properties also render it effective against convulsive coughs and asthma. It is an intestinal, pulmonary, and genitourinary antiseptic. Both the essence and crushed leaves are anti-venomous and, therefore, useful in treating insect and snake bites. Chewing thyme leaves soothes sore throats and tonsillitis. A handful of dried thyme boiled in a liter of water has been used as a hair tonic to halt and prevent hair loss. Finally, dried thyme used as a dentifrice strengthens the gums and dispels bad breath.

- Antibacterial and strong antiseptic.
- Expectorant and antispasmodic.
- Soothes sore throats and tonsillitis.
- Dispels bad breath.

Ylang-ylang

Cananga Odorata (Annonanceae)

The ylang-yang is an East Indian tree of the custard-apple family. It grows to be about sixty feet high, displaying magnificent, fragrant, yellowish green flowers.

The name of this tree translates as "flower of flowers." Certainly, the beautiful flowers, which smell like a mixture of almonds and jasmine, are its most impressive feature. The essence is obtained through steam distillation of these flowers. The oil is pale yellow, slightly bitter tasting, and very sweet smelling.

Ylang-yang has sedative, hypotensive, and euphoric actions on the nervous system. It is useful against anxiety, high blood pressure, and tension. Applications of this essence have reduced overaccelerated breathing and abnormally rapid heartbeats. Its antiseptic properties are particularly useful against intestinal infections.

This oil is a favorite for perfume—applied readily in its pure form, used as a fixative, or utilized as a bath oil to envelop the entire body in an exotic fragrance. As such, it is said to be an effective aphrodisiac. Because of its pleasant scent and soothing effect on the skin, ylang-ylang oil is widely used in facials, especially on oily complexions. But because the fragrance of ylang-ylang is so powerfully sweet, it should not be used in large doses for risk of inducing headaches or nausea.

- Sedates and induces euphoria.
- Said to be an effective aphrodisiac.
- Soothes the skin.
- Large doses cause headaches or nausea.

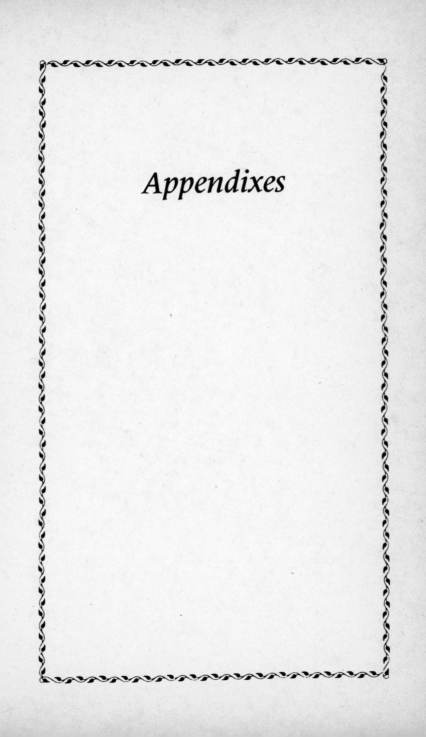

Appendixes

Perfume

THE WORD "PERFUME" COMES FROM LATIN; "PER" MEANS "through," and "fume" means "smoke." Although the word is Latin, perfumery itself is far older than the Roman Empire. The first perfumes were incense burned in religious ceremonies, as medicinal air fresheners meant to drive away evil spirits as well as germs, and as the follow-up to sexual intercourse. Perfume as we mean it today was exclusively an Oriental cosmetic for centuries. But aside from Asia, perfume figured everywhere in the ancient civilizations of Egypt, Greece, and Rome. In all of these cultures, men as well as women doused themselves in scent. Men rubbed scented oils on their beards, eyebrows, the soles of their feet, and, eventually, on handkerchiefs and stationery as well.

Alabaster jars of perfume—some still preserved!—have been found in the tombs of Egyptian pharaohs. Egyptians used perfume, namely cedarwood oil, to embalm their dead. Cleopatra was a walking perfumery; she anointed each part of her body with a different scent. For example, her feet were covered with aegyptium, a blend of almond oil, orange blossoms, honey, cinnamon, and henna; her hands were smeared with kyphi, an elaborate concoction including acacia, calamus, cassia, cinnamon, citronella, henna, juniper, myrrh, peppermint, and raisins! The barge upon which Cleopatra greeted Anthony was made of scented cedarwood, and incense burned all around her throne from dawn till dusk. Her elaborate perfumed baths provided the model for the famous Roman baths.

The Romans adored perfume. It was common in ancient Rome to coat the palm of one's hand with scented oils so that with a handshake one would transmit the scent and the friend or colleague would carry the memory of the meeting vividly with him. Romans were the first to apply perfume specifically to the wrists. Romans were obsessed with perfecting the art of public speaking, known as rhetoric; they realized that their scented wrists would send scent wafting in the air as they gesticulated, thereby helping them seduce the crowd. In the homes of royalty and the nobility, incense burned incessantly and flowers littered the bedchambers.

After the Fall of Rome, perfume moved eastward again. Only gradually did it—and hygiene in general—return to the West. The Crusaders brought perfume back to Europe during the thirteenth century. By the sixteenth century, perfumes were popular throughout Europe. During the Middle Ages, clothing was placed among bags scented in accordance with the season: in summer, roses, violets, and lilies were used; in winter, musk, aloe, and balsam. Sanitation conditions did not allow for frequent bathing—nor was bathing considered desirable. Most Europeans during this time considered the procedure unhealthy if indulged in more than once a month, and many abstained except for once a year; therefore, the practice of per-fumigating clothing was really essential! Medieval men and women commonly believed that the use of perfume caused the blood to move through the veins more energetically and the skin to glow. Because they used essential oils from plants as the constituents of their perfumes, to an extent this was probably true, as the research in the field of aromatherapy now demonstrates. During the Renaissance, Queen Elizabeth of England scented her gloves, cloak, and shoes daily. Reputedly, her favorite perfume was made from eight grams of musk placed in eight spoonfuls of rose water and a quarter of an ounce of sugar, which was then boiled for five hours and strained. Also during this period, dry sachets and perfumed lamps were crafted and sold by artisans. In the extravagant French court at Versailles, noblewomen were expected to wear a different scent virtually every day. Even during his military campaigns, Napoleon insisted on being well supplied with scented soaps and cases of eau de cologne. His wife, Josephine, was passionate about the scent of violet and she would cover her body with violet perfume in honor of Napoleon's triumphant returns home. One remnant of an early American contribution to the art of perfumery was manufactured by Caswell-Massey Company, Ltd., which claimed to be the "oldest chemists and perfumers in America." Its special fragrance, perhaps a forerunner of the contemporary classic Chanel No. 5, was simply called No. 6 Cologne.

Perfume is deeply entrenched with ritual religious practice. In ancient primitive cultures, resin, wood, and gum from intensely fragrant plants were burned in ceremonies. The high priests in Egypt were the first distributors of aromatics in that culture. And up until recently (and still today in special ceremonies), a cloud of fragrant incense would envelop most Catholic churches. The Bible, especially the Song of Solomon, is filled with references to scent. Even Mohammed encouraged his followers to use perfumes as a mark of holiness.

We share an attraction to perfume with other realms of nature: the plant, insect, and animal kingdoms. Our perfumes may not be as obvious as those of animals and plants, but we still use them to attract mates, mark our territories, and as a means of identification. It is interesting that for years some of the most coveted perfumes were secretions found in animal glands, for example, ambergris from the sperm whale, civet from the genital region of an Ethiopian cat, castoreum from the bellies of beavers, and musk taken from an East Asian deer. No one knows exactly how humans came to discover their attraction to these scents. However, we do know that the scent of musk, for example, literally produces hormonal changes in women: They develop shorter menstrual cycles and ovulate more frequently. This suggests why musk has come to be associated with masculine virility!

Luckily, most fragrances originally derived from animal substances are now produced synthetically, although some natural essences are still used as fixatives in perfumes. Regrettably, the use of natural plant essences has also virtually disappeared from the perfume industry. Only the most expensive ones are blended with natural essences. Synthetic chemicals, which are far less expensive to process, have been used extensively in perfumes since the nineteenth century. These synthetics are obtained chiefly from petrochemicals and coal tar. Sometimes essential oils from plants are used as a foundation for a perfume. Some plants whose oils are still used in the most expensive perfumes are rose, jasmine, lavender, cinnamon, patchouli, citronella, sandalwood, and rosemary.

In the United States, many synthetic substances have been developed to meet the rising demand for perfumes since many plants from which favorite essential oils are extracted are not native to this country. However, with the increasing interest in aromatherapy, many essential oils are now being imported.

Fragrant essences are found in the leaves, bark, wood, roots, and flowers, depending on the plant. The essential oils of a fragrant flower come from baglike structures called sacs. The process of extracting this oil from flower petals is delicate and costly. Three different methods are employed to accomplish this task:

1. Steam distillation. Steam is passed through the plant. The essential oil converts to gas that is then channeled through tubing, cooled, and returned to a liquid state.

2. Solvent extraction. Petals are dissolved in a solvent substance. This solvent is then removed, leaving behind a waxy residue containing the oil. The essential oil is then soaked in ethyl alcohol, causing it to rise to the top of the wax. With the application of heat, the alcohol evaporates and leaves a highly concentrated form of the essential oil.

3. Enfleurage. Flower petals are placed upon a layer of fat resting on a glass plate. The fat absorbs the oil from the petals. A greasy pulplike material forms, which is treated with alcohol, and then the oil is dissolved out.

Although most colognes and toilet waters are commonly referred to as perfumes, "true" perfumes are made with a higher concentration of extracted oil, which is why they are more expensive. True perfumes contain 10 to 20 percent essential oil dissolved in alcohol, while colognes have only 3 to 5 percent oil dissolved in 80 to 90 percent alcohol, with water constituting the balance. Toilet waters have only 2 percent perfume oil in 60 to 80 percent alcohol, while the balance is purified water.

Perfumery is a big business. But interestingly, 80 percent of the income generated by perfume industries comes from scented commodities—not human beings. Everywhere we go we are bombarded with scents, even if we don't acknowledge them: All household cleaners are scented; most chemical products are perfumed to mask their own, less pleasant smells; shopping malls release "pizza smell" through their air-conditioning vents to induce shoppers into their restaurants; scented air, carpet, linen, and clothing fresheners abound. Fragrance often has everything to do with the marketing success of a given product. If the aroma doesn't appeal, people won't buy it.

Perfumes have profound physiological and psychological effects on human beings. Smells seem able to release unconscious memories from childhood. Neurobiologists have demonstrated that work efficiency can be improved by introducing appealing perfumes into the work environment. But even with the impressive advances in medical research and technology, much about the mechanisms that trigger emotional responses to olfactory stimulation remain a mystery. Very little is known about the biological and chemical processes whereby humans distinguish one smell from another. We find it very difficult to describe perfumes in

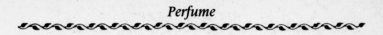

words. This is why the sense of smell has been called "the mute sense." In any case, it is universally recognized that the sense of smell is very powerfully entangled with human passions and behaviors. For confirmation, just note the names of some contemporary perfumes: Obsession, Passion, Tabu, Eternity, and Decadence. Furthermore, our lust for perfumes is ever seeking a new thrill. Perfumers are constantly developing new variations on older themes. With the exception of some natural fragrances, like essence of rose or jasmine, a "classic" perfume is one that survives for a decade. As a testimony to our scentophilia, today, in the United States alone, perfume is a billion-dollar-per-year industry.

Aromatic Literature:
Scent-sitive Art

"When from a long distant past nothing subsists, after the people are dead, after the things are broken and scattered, still, alone, more fragile, but with more vitality, more unsubstantial, more persistent, more faithful, the smell and taste of things remain poised a long time, like souls, ready to remind us, waiting and hoping for their moment, amid the ruins of all the rest; and bear unfaltering, in the tiny and almost impalpable drop of their essence, the vast structure of recollection."

MARCEL PROUST, *Remembrance of Things Past,*
"Swann's Way"

THE SENSE OF SMELL IS OFTEN CALLED THE MUTE SENSE because olfactory sensations are especially difficult to put into words. We tend to lapse into one of four modes when attempting to define a particular smell. In some instances, we resort to emotive adjectives—like "pleasant," "disgusting," or "warm"—that explain how a smell makes us feel.

We also tend to use vocabulary associated with other senses—like "musty," "robust," or "sweet"; this penchant is exemplified by these lines from Shakespeare's *Twelfth Night*: "It came o'er my ear like the sweet sound/That breathes upon a bank of violets." The third tendency is the use of tautological statements—like "Sandalwood oil has a woody fragrance." Finally, we often define one smell with another, such as this example from Archibald MacLeish's poem *Landscape As a Nude*: "The scent of her hair is of rain in the dust on her shoulders." Actually pinning a scent to the written page requires the combination of a vivid imagination and a sensitive nose. Thus, one of the tests of great literature is its ability to capture sensual pleasures (and horrors) within the confines of words.

The great literature of the Western world encourages us to be led by the nose. Homer depicts the bathing rituals of goddesses by exciting the nostrils: "Here first she bathes, and round her body pours/Soft oils of fragrance and ambrosial showers,/The winds, perfumed, the balmy gale conveys/Through heaven, through earth, and all the aerial ways"; Francis Thompson describes a purple rose as "a perfume press/whence the wind vintages/gushes of warmed fragrance, richer far/than all the flaverous ooze of Cyprus' vats"; Robert Herrick declares that his lover's body has "All the spices of the East... circumfused there"; Walt Whitman celebrates the smell of sweat, "aroma finer than prayer." Proust writes of limeflower tea and madeleines; James Joyce revels in baby urine and oilcloth; and Thoreau walks among max myrtle that smells "like small confectionery."

In the Old Testament's Song of Solomon, an extended declaration of love exchanged between a betrothed pair, drips with aromatic imagery. Because the young lovers are unable to act upon their physical desires they resort to a vivid, though euphemistic, poetic language. The verses alternate between the man and the woman:

> *While the king sitteth at his table, my spikenard sendeth forth the smell thereof.*
> *A bundle of myrrh is my well-beloved unto me; he shall lie all night betwixt my breasts.*
> *My beloved is unto me as a cluster of camphire in the vineyards of En-gé-di.*

> (1:12–14)

And later, the young man compares his beloved to a fragrant, enclosed garden:

> *Thy plants are an orchard of pomegranates, with pleasant fruits; camphire, with spikenard,*
> *Spikenard and saffron; calamus and cinnamon, with trees of frankincense; myrrh and aloes, with all the chief spices:*
> *A fountain of gardens, a well of living waters, and streams from Lebanon.*
> *Awake, O north wind; and come, thou south; blow upon my garden, that the spices thereof may flow out. Let my beloved come into his garden and eat his pleasant fruits.*

> (4:13–16)

There are few literary works more flagrantly fragrant and erotic. Another religious text, *The Prophet*, by Kahlil Gibran, uses comparisons to aromatic experience to describe spiritual behavior. Here is one example:

There are those who give with joy,
and that joy is their reward.
And there are those who give with pain,
and that pain is their baptism.
And there are those who give and know not
pain in giving, nor do they seek joy, nor
give with meanfulness of virtue;
They give as in yonder valley the myrtle
breathes its fragrance into space.
Through the hands of such as these God
speaks, and from behind their eyes he
smiles upon the earth.

This kind of metaphor concretizes something that would otherwise remain elusively abstract and intangible. In order to teach about moral values or metaphysical realms, all religious writers have had to utilize language rooted in our earthy, sensual experience. The paramount example of this tradition is the poetry of mystics, which, taken out of context, reads like passionate love poetry. But here is a passage from a fifteenth-century moralist who takes his metaphors to heart:

Also by odours this maie you learne,
Subtilness and groseness of matters to discerne.
A sweete-smelling thinge hath more puritie
and more of spirituall than stinking maie bee.
As colours changeth in your sight
So odours changeth the smelling by might.

THOMAS NORTON, *Ordinall of Alkimy*

Although his articulation is rather whimsical, it does seem that many writers share Norton's idea that foul smells and evil go hand in hand. In Shakespeare's *Hamlet*, Claudius, who murdered his brother in order to become king, says to himself: "O! my offense is rank, it smells to heaven" (III.iii.36). Milton depicts Satan as sniffing out carrion "Of carnage, prey innumerable . . . scent of living carcasses." During Prohibition in the United States, Irvin Shrewsbury Cobb described "corn licker" as follows: "It smells like gangrene starting in a mildewed silo." And in his *Inferno*, Dante offends the nose in creating his compelling portrait of the vilest thing of all: hell. In the third circle, where the gluttonous are punished, he tells us that they suffer thus: "Gross hailstones, water gray with filth, and snow/come streaking down across the shadowed air;/the earth, as it receives that shower, stinks" (Canto VI, 10–12). Throughout the ages artists have realized that the nose can help us understand other worlds—above and below.

Aside from taking us to realms outside of our mortal experience—places like hell and paradise—one way writers take us to the distant lands of this world is through their fragrant descriptions of landscapes. In the journal kept during his first voyage, one of Christopher Columbus's first comments, made in October of 1492, was "the air is soft as April in Seville, and it is a pleasure to be in it, so fragrant it is." In a more poetic rhapsody, D. H. Lawrence writes about New Mexico: "that lightness, that dry aromatic odor . . . one could breathe that only on the bright edges of the world, on the great grass plains or the sagebrush desert . . . Something soft and wild and free; something that whispered to the ear on the pillow, lightened the heart, softly, softly picked the lock, slid the bolts, and released the prisoned spirit of man into the wind, into the blue and gold, into the morning, into the morning!" At the other end of the spectrum, O. Henry in *A Municipal Report* describes another locale as follows: "Take of London fog 30 parts; malaria 10 parts; gas leaks 20 parts; dewdrops gathered in a brickyard at sunrise 25 parts; odor of honeysuckle 15 parts. Mix. The mixture will give you an approximate conception of a Nashville drizzle."

Arguably, the master of aromatic imagery is William Shakespeare. The extent to which Shakespeare used references to herbs and flowers in his poetry and plays has led many horticulturists to develop special "Shakespeare gardens" all around the world. In his play *The Winter's Tale*, Shakespeare gives to Perdita several pretty speeches with which she passes out flowers to the different characters visiting her sheep-shearing festival. She bestows her aromatic gifts based on what most becomes their "time of day." To the youths at the celebration she longs to give:

> *Daffodils,*
> *That come before swallow dares, and take*
> *The winds of March with beauty; violets, dim,*
> *But sweeter than the lids of Juno's eyes,*
> *Or Cythrea's breath; pale primroses,*
> *That die unmarried ere they can behold*
> *Bright Phoebus in his strength (a malady*
> *Most incident to maid); bold oxlips, and*
> *The crown imperial; lilies of all kinds,*
> *The flower-de-luce being one.*

(IV.iv.118–127)

In *A Midsummer Night's Dream,* Shakespeare depicts the scented woodland bedroom of the Fairy Queen, Titania, as follows:

> I know a bank whereon wild thyme blows,
> Where oxlips and the nodding violet grows;
> Quite overcanopied with luscious woodbine,
> With sweet musk roses, and with eglantine:
> There sleeps Titania, sometimes of the night,
> Lulled in these flowers with dances and delight.

> (II.ii.249–254)

In *The Tragedy of Antony and Cleopatra,* Shakespeare introduces his most sensual character in the following passage:

> The barge she sat in, like a burnished throne,
> Burned on the water; the poop was beaten gold,
> Purple the sails, and so perfumed, that
> The winds were love-sick with them.

> (II.ii.199–202)

Aside from these refined titillations of the nose, throughout his work Shakespeare devotes special attention to aromatic descriptions of a certain beverage, commonly called "sack" in his day and "the grape" in ours. In *Henry IV, Part 2,* Shakespeare's most famous tippler, Sir John Falstaff, claims that wine has the following impact on the nose: "It ascends me into the brain; dries me there all the foolish and dull and crudy vapours which environ it; makes it apprehensive, quick, forgetive, full of nimble, fiery, and delectable shapes; which delivered o'er to the voice, the tongue, which is the birth, becomes excellent wit" (IV.iii.97–102).

But Shakespeare is by no means alone in this venture. A special category of aromatic literature has been produced by and in response to viticulture. For connoisseurs, the character of a wine's "nose" is exceedingly important in determining its value. They have developed an elaborate language for identifying this nose. Wine bouquets have been described as "plumy, peppery, and high-toned," "attractive but earthy," "distinctive style and charm," "meaty but rather hard and wooden," "slightly vanilla with hints of oak and tobacco," or "an aura of opulent, crushed raspberries." To the uninitiated, descriptions of wine bouquets may sound comic or pretentious. However, scientists have confirmed that without a fragrance (or without a sense of smell with which to detect that fragrance) the taste of wine would be indistinguishable from that of water!

Many great writers have been conscious of the power of scent, and some have relied on olfactory experience to stimulate their creativity. Schiller, the eighteenth-century German poet and playwright, kept the top drawer of his writing desk filled with fresh apples. The French novelist Maupassant would sniff a bowl of strawberries soaking in ether as a means of overcoming writer's block. French philosopher Jean-Jacques Rousseau believed that the sense of smell was synonymous with the imagination.

With sufficient skill and sensitivity, literary artists can rouse the sense of smell and make readers putty in their hands. A recent example of such literature is, of course, Suskind's *Perfume*, which was mentioned earlier. By conjuring up olfactory memories an author can transport us to faraway lands, stir our deepest emotions, shower us in sensual delights, instruct, unnerve, repulse, arouse, and fulfill.

In a very legitimate sense, writing-through-the-nose keeps the past alive and nudges readers toward a fuller, more fragrance-conscious future.

Bibliography

Ackerman, Diane. *A Natural History of the Senses.* New York: Random House, 1990.

Amoore, J. E. *Nature.* 1967, 216:1084–87.

Bespaloff, Alexis. *The Fireside Book of Wine.* New York: Simon and Schuster, 1977.

Culpeper, Nicholas. *Culpeper's British Herbal,* enlarged 1850.

Erb, Russell C. *The Common Scents of Smell.* New York: World Publishing Co., 1968.

Gattefosse, Rene-Maurice. *Aromatherapie.* Paris: Girardot, 1928.

Hill, Madalene, and Barclay, Gwen. *Southern Herb Growing.* Fredericksburg, Tex.: Shearer Publishing, 1987.

Maury, Marguerite. *The Secret of Life and Youth.* 1964.

McKenzie, Daniel. *Aromatics of the Soul.* 1923.

Panati, Charles. *Extraordinary Origins of Everyday Things.* New York: Harper and Row, 1987.

Rovesti, Paolo. *Soap, Perfumery, and Cosmetics*. 1973, XLVI(8): 475–78.

Sanecki, Kay N. *The Book of Herbs*. Secaucus, N.J.: Chartwell Books, Inc.,

Shakespeare, William. *The Riverside Shakespeare*. Boston: Houghton Mifflin Co., 1974.

Suskind, Patrick. *Perfume*. New York: Alfred A. Knopf, Inc., 1986.

Tisserand, Robert B. *The Art of Aromatherapy*. Rochester, Vt.: Healing Arts Press, 1977.

Tompkins, Peter, and Bird, Christopher. *The Secret Life of Plants*. 1973.

Valnet, Jean. *The Practice of Aromatherapy*. Translated by Robin Campbell and Libby Houston. Rochester, Vt.: Healing Arts Press, 1989.